NEUROLOGICAL
CINEMATOGRAPHIC
ATLAS

NEUROLOGICAL CINEMATOGRAPHIC ATLAS

By S. PHILIP GOODHART, M.D.
PROFESSOR OF CLINICAL NEUROLOGY, COLUMBIA UNIVERSITY
CHIEF, NEUROPSYCHIATRIC DIVISION
MONTEFIORE HOSPITAL, NEW YORK

AND

BENJAMIN HARRIS BALSER, M.D.
MAJOR (MC)
ASSOCIATE IN NEUROLOGY, COLUMBIA UNIVERSITY
CONSULTANT IN NEUROPSYCHIATRY,
FIRST AIR FORCE, U.S. ARMY

KING'S CROWN PRESS
NEW YORK: MORNINGSIDE HEIGHTS
1944

COPYRIGHT 1944 BY
S. PHILIP GOODHART, M.D.
Printed in the United States of America

―――――

King's Crown Press is a division of Columbia University Press organized for the purpose of making certain scholarly material available at minimum cost. Toward that end, the publishers have adopted every reasonable economy except such as would interfere with a legible format. The work is presented substantially as submitted by the author, without the usual editorial attention of Columbia University Press.

FOREWORD

Of all neurologic diseases, those chiefly characterized by involuntary movements are perhaps the most difficult to grasp and classify. While some clinical entities among the dyskinesias are not rare—for example, the Parkinsonian syndrome, torticollis, athetosis, dystonia and Huntington's chorea—examples of them are often difficult to find in general hospitals, so that many students and practitioners do not have the opportunity of assimilating the range of symptoms which they display. Other types of dyskinesia, such as hepatolenticular degeneration, are almost curiosities, yet of great theoretical significance. Written descriptions of the dyskinesias are almost invariably thin and unsatisfactory—a rule to which Parkinson's famous essay forms a brilliant exception. Ordinary photographs seldom convey more than a fraction of the characteristic patterns of the movements

It is, therefore, particularly in the field of the dyskinesias that medical cinematography possesses its unique value. By its use, not only are the various movements seen in common and in rare conditions, portrayed as they might appear in a large clinic, but also the spectator has the opportunity to watch the evolution of the different varieties, to analyse the movements by means of "slow motion", and in many instances to see the results of special studies and even pathologic specimens, charts and diagrams, covering many years.

Dr. Goodhart and the late Dr. Frederick Tilney were among the pioneers in the field of neurologic cinematography, and some of the films in this collection are of historic interest. They have had an extraordinarily rich fund of material on which to draw at the Montefiore Hospital. The phenomena which are here presented should enable many who are less fortunately situated, to review rapidly and become familiar with the great range of symptomatology presented by the important group of dyskinesias. It is to be hoped further that a broadening and deepening of interest in the subject will lead eventually to an improved understanding of the mechanism of the activity of the damaged nervous system in such cases, and of the mechanism of the formation of the lesions. Given such knowledge, it is more than likely that methods will be found to arrest the progress of the destructive process or to alleviate the symptoms once they have become fixed. In no group of diseases is some form of relief more needed.

TRACY J. PUTNAM, M.D.

Columbia University, June, 1944

AUTHORS' PREFACE

The purpose of this manual, accompanying a series of 11 films demonstrating neurological subjects and produced by the authors, is to furnish detailed descriptions of the cases thus presented. The manual, therefore, is to be used in conjunction with the motion pictures. It is an endeavor to make available for critical observation, study, and particularly for medical instruction, groups of patients with various types of neurological diseases.

Our difficulties in the understanding of motor mechanisms, even in the lower forms of life, are infinitely magnified by a lack of comprehension and interpretative conception of vertebral motion in general, reaching its greatest complexity in man. Furthermore, the analysis and recording of different forms of motility are made more difficult by reason of the limitations and inadequacy of nomenclature as we endeavor to describe various forms of deformities of motion; the terms in general use are not only nondescriptive but lexicologically nondescripts of language when applied to clinical pathology.

Medical text-book descriptions, indeed even the demonstration of patients themselves with often necessarily lengthy and detailed histories, are apt to induce fatigue both in teacher and student. Subjects presented in animated pictorial forms are intensified in interest to the observer. The motion picture, with its exactness and brevity, is an asset in the teaching of neuropsychiatry to undergraduates and postgraduates, and in presentations of specific subjects before scientific gatherings. Furthermore, groups of patients showing, for example, various types of chronic chorea, Wilson's disease, etc., cannot ordinarily be immediately brought together for presentation. An atypical case for differential diagnosis, a chronological history of an instructive case, observed over a period of years, visualized in its progressive clinical features, cannot be accurately or graphically recorded in any way comparable to the visual presentation and graphic titular description of cinematographic reproduction.

Many years ago (1918), Dr. Frederick Tilney and Dr. Goodhart first demonstrated the value of the analysis of deformity of motion in nervous diseases by means of slow motion photography, the latter given the name, "Bradykinetic Analysis". This means of identifying and interpreting designs of abnormal motion has been utilized in the production of our films. The historical value and that of sequential record are well shown by the visually presented clinical signs in patients with postencephalitic deformities of motion, as observed during the epidemic following the World War. These cases were selected with especial reference to some unusual form of clinical manifestation.

AUTHORS' PREFACE

This small volume is to accompany the motion pictures. In each group a brief general outline of the disease entity precedes the description of the individual cases that follow. Thus demonstrator and student can become familiar with and follow the cases on the screen. For a number of years these films have been used and found most helpful in our courses for medical students of Columbia University. It is our endeavor to make them available for teaching purposes to medical groups and schools throughout the country.

As a knowledge of psychology and psychopathology is essential for the understanding of neuropsychiatric problems, it is evident that students in advanced psychology should be given instruction in the branch of medicine dealing with morbid mental and physical manifestations. Subtle relation between organic and psychogenic is one of growing practical and scientific interest. Therefore, a reel on psychosomatic disorders has been included in the series.

Since neuropsychiatry and endocrinology have so much in common, anatomically, physiologically and clinically, a reel presenting patients with somatic endocrine disorders has also been included. These were taken at an institution for mental defectives.

Abnormal neurological conditions associated with pathological signs relating to vision are demonstrated in a reel indexed as "Neuro-ophthalmological Conditions".

This work was done at the Montefiore Hospital and its publication made possible by a specific grant from the United Hospital Fund.

CONTENTS

Chorea	1
Convulsive and Allied Conditions	5
Dystonia Musculorum Deformans	8
Epidemic Encephalitis	19
Friedreich's Hereditary Ataxia	27
Little's Disease and Double Athetosis	29
Muscular Dystrophies, Atrophies and Allied Conditions	31
Progressive Hepato-lenticular Degeneration	42
Neuro-ophthalmological Conditions	46
Psychoneuroses—Organic Signs—Their Differentiation	50
Somatic Endocrine Types	54
Encephalographic Studies in Extrapyramidal Diseases	61
Appendix	63

CHOREA

(Film running time: 10 minutes)

Chorea, a generic term meaning "dance," appears in two more or less distinct and yet, in motor expression, clinically similar entities, namely as an acute disease, known as Sydenham's chorea, and as a chronic affection. The latter group is subdivided into types with especial reference to etiology and with associated specific pathology.

The acute and the variants in the chronic types are both characterized by very similar deformities of motion. In the chronic, the abnormal movements are of slower tempo, though very similar in design.

The age of onset, etiology, course and prognosis are very different in the two groups.

Visually studied by means of "slow motion" photography, the movements in the chronic group are revealed as apparently unconscious yet of purposeful design and meaning. Grossly observed, they are involuntary, somewhat clownish, graceful or playful and non-repetitive in the same form; again they are brief, explosive and unsustained and not completed. Facial grimacing, sudden respiratory and explosive articulatory fragments and grunts, with difficulty in articulation, mastication and swallowing are often seen in varying combination and degree in this rather grotesque clinical entity. A halting, lurching, clownish design gives character to the gait.

Involvement of the intellectual and emotional spheres, as occurs in both acute and chronic progressive chorea, is referred to under the serial forms sketched briefly as follows:

CHRONIC TYPES

1. *Huntington's*—A hereditary familial disease characterized by abnormal involuntary movements. Age of onset is usually between 35 and 45; often associated with a psychotic state and mental deterioration. Its course is progressive. Gradual, progressive mental deterioration is a prominent feature. Emotional, delusional and deteriorative symptoms vary in individual cases, probably determined by biological variants in the ancestry and personality.

2. *Arteriosclerotic*—No evidence of hereditary influence; onset usually somewhat sudden, between 40 and 55 years, with evidence of generalized arteriosclerosis. The movements may be general or limited to one

extremity or to one-half of the body (monochorea, hemi-chorea). The mental state is a variable one; there may be mild psychotic symptoms and mental deterioration.

3. *Senile*—The onset is in the senium and is gradual and slowly progressive. The involuntary movements are generalized and usually of mild degree; mental symptoms other than those of senescence are not present.

4. *Postencephalitic*—Heredity is not a factor. The patient has, at some time in the past, suffered from an acute attack of encephalitis, usually of the epidemic type. The onset may occur at any age.

Pathology—In the chronic types the following pathological changes have been found:
- a. Leptomeningitis affecting predominantly the area of the frontal lobes.
- b. Atrophy, usually of the frontal lobes, sometimes limited to a few convolutions and again generalized.
- c. Dilation of the ventricular system.
- d. Degenerative cell changes in the basal ganglia affecting especially the small cells of caudate and putamen.
- e. Progressive gliosis in the involved areas.
- f. Pathological changes in the coats of the arterial walls (i.e. externa, media, intima).

ACUTE SYDENHAM'S CHOREA

A disease entity, also clinically characterized by irregular involuntary contraction of groups of muscles, gives rise to deformities of motion very similar to those of the chronic progressive degenerative form; it is probably of the nature of an acute infection occurring in young people. It is usually attended by psychic disturbance in the emotional sphere and frequently associated with acute endocarditis and the rheumatic diathesis. It is most common between the ages of five and fifteen years; females are affected in greater ratio. The movements in the acute form are more rapid than in the chronic and may involve one or more segments as well as head, trunk and muscles of articulation, mastication and deglutition. The onset is often preceded by a mild state of irritability and emotional upset. The deep reflexes may sometimes be absent or difficult to elicit and there is often hypotonia.

Though the prognosis for the acute episode is favorable, the disease is often recurrent.

The following cases illustrate the various types of chorea. The patients were selected with a view to demonstrating characteristic clinical features. The chronic group includes Huntington's, arteriosclerotic, senile and postencephalitic types; the acute is illustrated by a case of Sydenham's chorea.

Case 1—40 years of age, Huntington's type. The movements are those seen in the early stages of this disease.

Case 2—49 years of age, Huntington's chorea. The first symptoms were observed at the age of 35. The heredo-familial factor, characteristic of the Huntington type, is emphasized by the fact that the father and a brother suffered from the same illness as the patient. Delusional ideas and intellectual deterioration appeared early and progressed with the somatic symptomatology. All segments of the body, including the facial muscles, became involved. One observes the involuntary, purposeless, extensive movements which are apparently without pattern and are nonrepetitive in exact form. They are "clownish" and include facial grimacing. Like all movements of similar pathology, they cease during sleep.

Case 3—44 years of age, Huntington's chorea. A sister was similarly afflicted. As in the preceding case, there was a gradual mental deterioration concomitant with the dyskinesia. The latter, though less in degree, is of the same form as in the preceding case. Observations of the patient, made four years later, show progression in mental deterioration and dyskinesia. This is, in a measure, revealed in a study of the picture. She finally required assistance in walking because of the interference with voluntary coordinated movements.

Case 4—45 years of age, Huntington type. Early in her illness, she became psychotic to a degree which required hospitalization; she had dominating persecutory delusions. The clinical picture was apparently precipitated by an intense emotional upset. It may be observed that the dyskinesias are less extensive than usually seen.

Case 5—50 years of age, belongs to the arteriosclerotic group. He developed delusional trends and, later, marked mental deterioration. The movements approach a tic-like design.

Case 6—62 years of age, also belongs in the arteriosclerotic group. The configuration of the abnormal movements is characteristic of chronic degenerative chorea.

Case 7—62 years of age, arteriosclerotic type. The pictures of this patient delineate the clownish design of some of the movements in this disease. Observe how the pattern of normal gait is distorted. In the performance of the finger to finger and finger to nose tests, note the distortion due to interference with the execution of normal voluntary movements. In the supine position there is a form of muscular activity in the lower extremities which is suggestive of "progression movements."

Case 8—30 years of age, her illness followed soon after acute epidemic encephalitis. The dyskinesias are most extensive. The clinical picture more closely approximates that of the fully developed chronic degenerative chorea.

Case 9—29 years of age, an early case of chorea of encephalitic etiology. The kinetic defects are more clearly brought out when finer movements are attempted, such as walking in a direct line, one foot successively in front of the other. A fragment of the encephalitic clinical pathology remains as myoclonic movements in both quadriceps femoris muscle groups. Films of this patient are also shown demonstrating the marked progress of the disease in later years.

Case 10—28 years of age, postencephalitic type. These pictures were taken with a slow motion camera in order to analyze the dyskinesias; their study reveals elements of both dystonia musculorum deformans and chronic degenerative chorea.

Case 11—38 years of age, postencephalitic type. The first symptoms appeared during the 3rd month of her pregnancy. These pictures were taken simultaneously at regular speed and also with a slow motion camera. The disturbances of motility in this patient are characteristic of chronic degenerative chorea. An analysis of the pictures, as studied in slow motion, suggests a purposive element in these apparently purposeless movements.

Case 12—19 years of age. This is a case of acute chorea, Sydenham type. The movements are more rapid but in design are strikingly like those in the chronic degenerative type.

CONVULSIVE AND ALLIED CONDITIONS

(Film running time: 11 minutes)

These reels present a group of cases of convulsive and allied conditions. An analysis of each type is made to clarify the points of differentiation between them with special reference to their etiology. Included are the following: generalized tic or maladie des tics, generalized myoclonic movements following acute epidemic encephalitis, myoclonus epilepsy (Unverricht), palatal myoclonus, catalepsy, narcolepsy associated with cataplexy, convulsive state in hypoglycemia, Jacksonian seizures (due to cerebral neoplasm), convulsions of psychogenic origin.

Case 1—12 years of age, shows a characteristic clinical picture of *generalized tics*. There is a repetition in design of movement in the same groups of muscles. The convulsive tic is a sudden, explosive, automatic one, and is accompanied by a brief sharp outcry. There is no alteration in consciousness and no other abnormal psychic or physical signs. There is no intellectual defect.

Case 2—60 years of age, shows *generalized tics* existing in later life. Observe involvement of some of the facial, left shoulder girdle and left pectoral muscles. The psychogenic characteristic of this entity is emphasized by analysis of the postural elements of the gait. There is no alteration in consciousness or intellectual defect.

Case 3—13 years of age, passed through a severe illness, namely, acute epidemic encephalitis, two years before these pictures were taken. As residua, are the generalized violent *myoclonic movements* seen here; both agonists and antagonists are involved. The movements, although incessant throughout the day, do not give rise to pain. As observed 18 months later, the movements become markedly less and changed in character; they are less violent and less extensive and the patient has some voluntary control over them; they are more "choreiform" in design. As somatic symptoms regressed, the patient developed behavior disorders; she became irritable, aggressive and showed paranoid tendencies, necessitating her removal to a mental hospital.

Case 4—26 years of age, of Italian parentage, is a case of *myoclonus epilepsy*. This comparatively rare entity appears to establish some relationship between two major motor disorders—the convulsive state and myoclonia. In myoclonus epilepsy, as designated by Unverricht, a familial affection, convulsive seizures gradually develop; the attacks are finally recovered from while myoclonic movements persist. This case shows the intimate relationship between these two forms of motor disorder. In this patient a generalized convulsive seizure may be induced by an irritating stimulus, in this instance in the form of inhalation of ammonium hydroxide, as demonstrated in the picture. The myoclonic movements are constant; observe the involvement of muscles of the extremities, especially the upper and left lower, and the frontalis portion of the occipitofrontalis muscles. Transitional and abortive states are reported in literature.

Case 5—A patient 49 years of age who formerly suffered from generalized convulsions with unconsciousness, now presents typical myoclonic movements confined to the head and trunk musculature; this is another case of *myoclonus epilepsy*. In this patient, the movements, more or less constant, may be accentuated by such stimuli as a sudden loud noise or flash of light.

Case 6—51 years of age, suffers from diffuse vascular disease of the brain including the brain stem. The especial feature demonstrated here is *myoclonic movement of the soft palate;* its pathology is doubtless within the brain stem. Observe also the involvement of structures controlling eye-movements.

Case 7—19 years of age, presents the entity known as *catalepsy*. The incidental mild defect in gait is due to poliomyelitis suffered in childhood. The picture of catalepsy consists of sudden spontaneous falling, attended by momentary rigidity, especially of the flexors of the extremities. Careful observation of the pictures presented discloses what may be termed "abortive" attacks; in these, the patient, about to fall, gains sufficient voluntary control to enable him to maintain the upright posture. Consciousness is not affected.

Case 8—31 years of age, presents the syndrome of *narcolepsy associated with cataplexy*. In the pictures the patient is seen to suddenly fall as though in a state of collapse. Consciousness is lost for a variable period, usually for about 30 to 60 seconds. As shown in the preceding patients, in cases of catalepsy there is momentary muscular rigidity with no interference in consciousness; in narcolepsy, with cataplexy, there is general-

CONVULSIVE AND ALLIED CONDITIONS

ized muscular flaccidity with loss of consciousness. In both, the patient suddenly falls to the ground. The last two entities are clinically placed in the group of the epilepsies.

Case 9—47 years of age, suffers from periodic, spontaneous, *hypoglycemic episodes*. In these attacks, abnormal motor, as well as psychic manifestations, are seen; there is an apparent inter-relationship between the two. One sees bizarre forms of gait and attitude; they rapidly change from one design to another; some of the patterns suggest simple purposeful activity and are much like the "picking and groping" seen in patients with pathology of the frontal lobes. They are also suggestive of the seemingly automatic movements (equivalents) of convulsive states and are also seen in organic delirium. The evanescent, fleeting character of the patterns indicates the absence of fixed organic pathology and strongly suggests that the basic pathological process is bio-chemical or physiological in origin. There is a lowering of the threshold of consciousness and the patient's contact with her environment is superficial.

Case 10—48 years of age, was operated upon for glioblastoma multiforme of the right fronto-parietal lobes. Surgical removal was followed by recurrence leaving the present demonstrable signs. The *seizures are Jacksonian* in type and involve the left half of the body; they are initiated by a turning of the head and trunk to the right, in tonic spasm, followed by typical clonic movements in the same segments. As is not unusual, the facial musculature is not involved; there is clouding of consciousness during the attacks. The cause of these seizures is the mechanical effect of the tumor upon the right motor cortical areas.

Case 11—47 years of age. The complete psychogenic syndrome of this patient is depicted in another reel among the cases demonstrating hysteria. The phase showing the convulsive type of movement is presented here for comparison with the convulsive seizures of organic etiology. These movements were the motor components in the expression of an episode induced by an emotional upset.

DYSTONIA MUSCULORUM DEFORMANS

(Film running time: 20 minutes)

Studies of this disease are presented. The basic characteristic feature is the alternating play of hyper- and hypotonus of the groups of muscles involved. There are two recognized types, the kinetic and the static. In the former, one sees various designs in movement of the bodily segments, depending upon the groups of muscles involved. Among the various forms of distorted movement are torsion spasms of the head, neck, shoulder, and pelvic girdle, trunk and upper and lower extremities; in the hand and foot this produces a typical movement and posture of pronation and adduction of the hand and plantar flexion and adduction of the foot. In the static type, these postures may become fixed. From the standpoint of etiology, two forms are recognized: the idiopathic, with its first signs usually appearing in the years of puberty; the encephalitic, as a sequel to the acute disease. Other names given this clinico-pathological entity are dysbasia lordotica progressiva, torsion spasm and tortipelvis.

Presented first in this reel is a case of encephalitic origin, which was studied from its incipiency to the demise of the patient, a period of seventeen years; post-mortem studies were made. Both the clinical history and the pathological findings are graphically shown in the pictures. Patients are then shown illustrating the various forms of dystonia with their individual signs, and the progress of the disease.

Case 1—This patient came under observation at 16 years of age. The onset of the disease was apparently sudden and followed an experience attended by fright and emotional upset; she sought safety in flight by running, almost to exhaustion, during a severe electrical storm. Shortly afterward, there appeared bizarre movements in both upper and lower extremities. In the early observation and studies of this case, organic etiology was given but little consideration; the movements, attitudes, and the emotional state of the patient suggested a psychogenic entity. As one studies the pictures in retrospect, analyzing some of the early kinetic features, one now would interpret them as bearing significant designs of organic pathology. On the basis of the diagnosis of psychoneurosis, various forms of intensive psychotherapy were applied at the onset. As the pictures unfolded a fully developed organic syndrome, therapeutic measures, consisting of prolonged application of plaster casts and medication were instituted.

This case brings up for study the important subtle relationship between what has been termed the psychogenic, as distinct from disease entity of recognized organic pathology. Can a psychogenic pattern be crystallized into a fixed organic design? Were there no psychogenic precursor in the situation, would the organic entity have been one of dystonia musculorum deformans? We feel that this case tends to confirm the opinion that there is definite and intimate relationship in character between early psychogenic states and the subsequent development of organic disease. Does one, in some cases, at first see only the shadow of a developing pathology? Does the plastic design become a fixed, an organized mould, and is the determining factor a variable component based upon the patient's inherent reactions? The pathology of dystonia musculorum deformans has been established as being at the sensori-motor level of the basal ganglia; it may be suggested, that psychopathological activity is at that same (anatomical) level.

Some of the scenes were taken with two synchronously operating cameras, one in slow motion and the other in normal tempo. The initial gross movements of the extremities conform to no organic design; the posture and gait are those of astasia abasia. Only in slow motion is a peculiar, wave-like movement of the muscles of the thigh visually demonstrated. We have characterized this movement as "vermicular". These movements are not recognizable by palpation, nor are they visible to the naked eye. This unique finding in the analysis of muscular activity is probably the clinical analogue of athetotic movement, and the microscopic pathology is that form of finer tissue change, known as status marmoratus and status dysmyelinisatus of the corpus striatum.

The patient is shown seated in a wheelchair at an early stage of the illness. The design of the involuntary movements in the feet is distinctly that of the typical "dystonic foot". Visualize this foot in fixation and you have the classical "dystonic foot". It is a fact however, that in purely functional conditions, one sometimes sees the same design of posture. Movements of the upper extremities are clearly visualized in the successive pictures.

Plaster casts were applied to both lower extremities, partly to give support, but more particularly for the purpose of restricting the abnormal movements of the feet and thus to maintain a more normal posture. This simple restriction of movement produced, as you observe on the screen, such a change in the patient's affective display as to indicate a marked psychogenic component. Note the cheerfulness of the patient and apparent cessation of abnormal movement as she reacts to this simple procedure. Pictures taken ten months later reveal a bizarre posture of the feet, a combination of "dystonic foot" with strong suggestion of a psychogenic element. The "vermicular wave" in the leg, persisting at this time, is more grossly demonstrated.

The patient was discharged from the hospital and the clinical picture remained essentially unchanged for about four years. She then suddenly developed symptoms that were doubtless due to involvement of the sympathetic nervous system. These symptoms appeared as episodes of gastro-intestinal upset; periods of violent vomiting and abdominal distention culminated in one very severe attack, in which a surgical abdominal condition was diagnosed and she was removed to a hospital. Spontaneous, somatic, dystonic features unfolded. Her abdominal signs and symptoms were due to involvement of central vegetative nerve centers (hypothalamus) as part of the organic syndrome—dystonia. Periodic episodes of this type occurred during the latter years of her illness. She was then readmitted to the Montefiore Hospital. Pictures taken shortly afterward disclose typical dystonic deformities of posture and movement, characteristic of dystonia musculorum deformans. Her mental attitude, suggesting a euphoric state, was in marked contrast to her extensive somatic involvement. For many years thereafter, this affective display continued in spite of advancing physical discomfort. Observe in the pictures the strong flexor fixation of the lower extremities, the dystonic posture of the hands and feet—fingers flexed, hands strongly pronated and torsion spasm of the trunk and pelvis. Attempts to overcome the static hypertonicity in the lower extremities give rise to intense pain. There is an occasional typical interplay of tone—hyper and hypo- between agonist and antagonist groups of muscles.

The patient was placed under anesthesia and studies made of its effect upon the deformities and distortions of movement. With the patient completely under its influence, one sees total relaxation of the groups of muscles formerly in strong contracture. As the effects of the anesthetic pass off, there is a synchronous return to the preceding abnormal postures. These studies enable one to draw conclusions concerning the influence of the cerebral cortex upon the extrapyramidal system. The relationship between the depth of anesthesia and the expression of extrapyramidal activity is shown in the interplay, as the degree of anesthesia is varied.

A sudden and remarkable change of posture occurred on one occasion during the night, as is shown in the pictures; it was followed within a few days by a return to the characteristic dystonic posture. This rare design and the rapidity of transformation are suggestive of a purely psychogenic origin.

The patient was again anesthetized to overcome the deformities and induce complete relaxation, so that plaster casts could be applied. After wearing the casts for several months, she is again shown immediately following removal of the casts. The patient's facial expressions of pain at this time are due to the tendency of the lower extremities to return at once to the patterns which characterize the clinical pathology of dystonia. Physical therapy was applied in an effort to maintain what had been accomplished by the use of casts. This treatment was effective for a few months only and then the former deformities of posture reappeared and strong sedatives were required for the relief of the painful, progressive contractures.

The patient remained under observation in the hospital for the next ten years. The clinical picture remained essentially the same except for recurrent episodes of severe autonomic disturbance, characterized by bouts of intractable vomiting, hiccoughing and gastro-intestinal paresis and distension. Various forms of therapy, medicinal and mechanical, proved of no avail and finally, constant sedation was required for the patient's comfort. Death was due to asthenia and cardiac failure.

In a case similar in many respects to this one and shown in another reel, pronounced improvement has continued for over seven years following the repeated application of plaster casts; the patient became ambulatory and was able to leave the hospital and return to work.

Case 2—Boy, 13 years of age, is first shown in the supine position. Essentially all groups of muscles are involved with the resulting characteristic type of involuntary movement. The phase of hypertonicity varies in its duration; for example, the ilio-psoas and quadriceps femoris groups of the right lower extremity at times remain in a state of tonic contraction for a few seconds, producing flexion at the hip and extension at the knee. Observe the movements in the right hand and forearm, in design assuming the characteristic posture of the static type. Note the involvement of the sternocleidomastoids producing transient torticollis. Some of the muscular contractions are so strong and extensive as to induce gross bodily deformity. Volition plays no role in these movements. This boy died at 16 years of age, of acute dilatation of the stomach. Post-mortem studies revealed extensive pathology in the hypothalamic nerve centers of the diencephalon. While the hypothalamic areas of the brain are frequently involved, rarely does one see complete paralysis of the gut. The stomach was enormously dilated and appeared as a huge sack reaching from the diaphragm to the pelvis.

Case 3—This case, idiopathic in origin, was studied with two cameras operating synchronously, one to produce slow motion and the other normal speed pictures; the postural designs are thus more clearly delineated. Patient is first shown seated and then in walking. To this bizarre but distinctive design of gait and posture, the name "dromedary" has been applied and the extremely high arched foot designed as "semilunar foot".

The trunk and foot deformities are the result of static fixation; the movements of the head, dystonic in design, suggest fragmental torticollis.

Case 4—The pictures of this patient were taken at various intervals over a period of nine years. During this time the various therapeutic measures consisted of the application of plaster casts and surgical intervention. As in all these cases, medication had little and only temporary effect; surgical measures likewise proved futile. As is usual in these cases, the movements themselves are not painful or exhausting. However, the constant muscular activity causes true physiological hypertrophy and, as in all cases, prolonged effort by the patient to voluntarily overcome the dystonic movements gives rise to intense fatigue.

The first pictures show the patient with the typical deformities of posture and movement involving all segments of the body including the head components. The patient cannot stand or walk without assistance. There is an evanescent torticollis; the right leg, flexed at the knee, assumes this static posture for a variable period, due to a prolonged phase of hypertonus of the hamstring group; the left foot momentarily assumes the arched dystonic posture. Now and then the torsion spasm of the pelvis becomes evident; in another phase one sees extreme lordosis, almost to a degree of opisthotonus.

The next pictures were taken four years later. A plaster cast embracing practically the entire body had been previously applied and allowed to remain for three months; she was thereafter given massage to the wasted muscles. One now sees a tendency to the static type; lordosis, tilting of pelvis, sustained torticollis are present. This case presents, at this time, one of the prominent features often seen early in dystonia, namely, a tendency to walk on the ball of the foot. In the early cases this feature is not as marked as in this patient. One can appreciate how intense the central stimulus must be to produce such a high degree of hypertonicity in the neck muscles giving the marked deformity, causing the head to be so strongly held in lateral flexor-rotary position. We call attention to these specific postures since they characterize the various phases of dystonia musculorum deformans. Fragments, pathognomonic of this entity, are seen in every case, in one form or another.

This patient was operated upon shortly after her admission to Montefiore Hospital. A bilateral anterior column cordotomy was performed and, at the same time, crushing of anterior and posterior cervical second, third and fourth nerve roots. The effects, including local sensory changes, were temporary; essentially no influence on the dystonic movements was observed. Five years later another surgical procedure was tried; spinal accessory nerves and cervical first, second and third anterior and posterior roots were resected bilaterally. The final pictures show the patient after this procedure. The dystonic movements were still uninfluenced; the sternocleidomastoid and trapezius muscles continued in their alternately hyper- and hypotonic states. Strangely enough, there appeared to be little or no effect upon the motor innervation of these muscles. Apparently one must look to the sympathetic nervous system in the production of these movements.

The difficulties of complete section of all of the anterior roots of the spinal accessory nerve for torticollis are familiar. Before considering the influence of the sympathetic nervous system in the production of dystonic movements, one must be certain that the surgical section of pyramidal, extra-pyramidal and peripheral pathways has been complete.

Case 5—Before her acute illness (epidemic encephalitis) this girl was a professional toe dancer. There is some degree of psychogenic superimposition or rather integration of personality and of, more or less, "conditioned" volition. However, the organic elements are manifest and one observes dystonic fragments—hyper-and hypotonicity, as well as evidence of cerebellar components in the bizarre picture.

Case 6—In its early stage location is limited to the neck muscles and upper extremities. The dystonic features are outstanding and confined to the upper half of the body.

Case 7—Shows a picture of a reversed so-called Magnus DeKleign design of posture. This represents a distinct postural relationship between the muscle groups of the upper extremities and those of the head and neck muscles. As observed in the static types, the fixed posture is determined by the hypertonicity as it gives fixation to the postural design. These last two cases suggest that there is definite localization in the extrapyramidal system.

Case 8—This patient demonstrates a static type of dystonia. The condition has remained unchanged for some twenty-five years. Observe the sardonic expression of the facies. Involvement of the facial muscles is very rare. In this very unusual clinical picture, all groups of voluntary muscles are involved in static fixation.

Case 9—19 years of age, is a classical case of the static type of dystonia. She shows the characteristic postural deformities of trunk and extremities. The head and arms are fixed in extreme extension, the legs flexed at the knees and hips and the hands and feet are in distinctive posture. There are almost imperceptible hyper- and hypotonic contractions of the various muscle groups.

Case 10—12 years of age, is a case of the kinetic type of dystonia, of encephalitic origin; involvement is limited to the left lower extremity. The foot is of dystonic design and the interplay of hypo- and hypertonus is exquisitely demonstrated in the quadriceps femoris group. In side view, the muscles of the thigh are seen in their transitory state of sudden contraction.

Case 11—This patient suffered from acute epidemic encephalitis about one year previous to the first pictures which were taken in 1922. She is shown seated and presents the classical kinetic type of dystonia. There are generalized typical muscle group contractions and one of the deformities seen is a fragmentary evanescent torticollis.

Same patient is shown 12 years later (1934). Shortly after these pictures were taken, she suffered from episodes of involvement of the vegetative nervous system; she had a series of gastro-intestinal disturbances at irregular periods, associated with emotional upsets, the former so severe that she became emaciated and bedridden. Typical postural deformities developed, as seen in the static type of dystonia. Series of plaster casts were applied over a period of about one year and there was gradual improvement in the clinical picture, as is evident in the scene now shown. The left leg is held in extension and the right upper extremity shows the distinctive postural elements of dystonia. Observe that, at this time, the normal associated movements are partially suppressed in both upper extremities, more so on the right.

The final scenes were taken four years later (1938). The development of a Parkinsonian syndrome is evident. There is now complete loss of associated movements in both upper extremities; gait, posture and facies are classically Parkinsonian. The value of a mild degree of corrective support for the deformed parts is strikingly demonstrated by the contrast, as shown when the patient walks with and without the aid of shoes. Her physical limitations at this time did not prevent her from engaging in remunerative occupation after discharge from the hospital; she resumed her vocation of dressmaking. The usual trunkal deformities are conspicuously absent here, as shown in the maintained normal configuration of the spine.

Case 12—14 years of age, presents an interesting segmental distribution of muscle group involvement in dystonia. He shows both kinetic and static forms with involvement limited to structures above the pelvis. There is fixed torticollis and tortipelvis. The posture, attitude and movements in this case are in their entirety unusual, but present classical elements of dystonia.

Case 13—13 years of age, a case of idiopathic dystonia, is shown within a few months of onset of the illness. The kinetic features are outstanding; the gradual transformation of the kinetic to segmental static form is shown in the design of the left leg. Although there is no motor weakness, the patient's inability to walk is apparently due to the loss of the pattern and design constituting the elements of gait. The patient is shown suspended; the movements continue in the same form, thus demonstrating their independence of the "body-righting" reflexes. Death came suddenly due to acute dilatation of the stomach. It is of interest to note that in a dystonia patient, a boy of 15 shown previously, a similar enormous gastric dilatation suddenly occurred and was the immediate cause of death.

Cases 14, 15 and 16—Three cases of familial dystonia musculorum deformans, a brother and his two sisters.

In this family group of dystonia musculorum deformans each member presents a different degree of severity and progress of the disease. The family stock was recorded as having been substantially without taint except in one important particular; on the paternal side there is a more or less direct history of dystonia, in that the father's sister and her daughter were afflicted with a disease similar to that of the three patients here described. The brother is the least afflicted of the group. As in the case of the sisters, his early life up to the time of onset of the present illness was quite normal. The motor disturbance began in his 13th year, and as in the case of the younger sister, manifested itself especially in any attempt at execution of finer movements with the right hand, e.g. writing. The patient is intelligent and from the first made every effort to overcome his difficulty. He fully realized the progress and serious deformity which the disease had shown in his sisters and was fearful, even before the onset of his illness, that he, too, might become a sufferer. Indeed, the boy made unusual efforts by exercise and intense mental endeavor to maintain control over the affected upper extremities; he continued with great determination as he felt the right leg, more particularly the right foot, assume spasmodic, uncontrollable, involuntary attitudes in attempting movement.

The cinematographic representation of his gait shows a sudden external rotation of the foot and spontaneous flexion at the knee and hip with inward rotation at the hip. In normal projection, as he runs, a limp is seen. Slow motion photography (bradykinetic analysis) shows a partial failure of coordinate time reaction, in groups of agonists and antagonists. A study of our series of dystonias shows this failure as a feature in all cases. For example, the forceful hyperextension of the foot, common to all of the cases of dystonia, appears as a failure in the time limitation of the muscular contraction, or, in other words, an excessive overflow of innervation (hypertonia). The peculiar character of this kinetic overflow in the agonist groups differentiates the organic from the functional disease, with which this latter spasmodic condition has often been confused.

The slight rotation of the thigh seen on normal projections, together with a raising of the foot in equinus position and flexion at the knee and hip, is, in reality, a widespread disorganization of the motor elements of gait. The extreme pronation of the right upper extremity gives the characteristic posture which in the more advanced stages assumes fixation. The torsion of the pelvis, commonly described in this disease, is only suggested in this patient, though a study in slow motion of the long muscles of the back and those about the pelvis shows the tendency to rotary motion.

In a study, by bradykinetic analysis, of the individual muscle groups in this patient, those of the right thigh stand out with abnormal intensity during periods which require their function only to a slight degree, thus indicating hyperkinetic innervation. This appears as a prolongation of muscular action; in less degree, this is also conspicious in the left thigh. It may be suggested that this overflow is an incipient phase of the characteristic deformities seen in the dystonias.

A sister, an intelligent girl of 18, was the second in this family of three to become a victim of dystonia. Her condition represents a degree of involvement between that of the slightly affected brother and the more advanced case of another sister. There was no retardation in early development, the three children of this family having begun to walk and talk before the age of two.

When twelve years of age, the patient noticed a sudden jerking or forced movement, in the form of pronation, beginning in the right hand. This motor difficulty showed definite advance in the performance of skilled movements generally, particularly in writing, and there were peculiar stiffening and worm-like movements in the fingers which seemed to extend suddenly upon attempts to grasp objects; this suggests an athetotic element. The left hand soon became similarly affected. Pathological findings in dystonia show much of the same kind of structural changes (status marmoratus and status dysmyelinisatus), as found in athetosis. Within a few months the right leg showed some disturbance of motility. Gradually a feeling of tension developed in the leg, the extremity became flexed and the hip more or less fixed in this position. As in all of these cases of dystonia musculorum deformans, this patient became easily exhausted upon attempts at voluntary movements requiring resistance to the opposing dystonic muscle groups. This is doubtless due in large measure to the efforts at suppression and the extra endeavor to use muscle groups, some of which are already involved. The relation of the trunk and the pelvis is such as to cause lordosis of the lower dorsal and lumbar spines, and the entire body assumes an attitude of emprosthotonos. The characteristic hyperextension (plantar flexion) of the foot is present and a limp much more pronounced than in the brother. There is a marked likeness in the general postural design of the three members of this group.

In this patient, fixation developed at the knee and the hip. The hyperstatic condition is also seen in the inward rotation of the knee as well as in the marked plantar flexion of the foot and the toes. When studied by means of slow motion pictures the hyperkinetic overflow becomes evident in the soleus-gastrocnemius groups. Fixation at the hip restricts extension, so that the trunk is not projected to the usual degree and in the characteristic manner.

The third case of the series is the most advanced of the three children in this family. The patient is a young woman, twenty years of age. Her condition is the result of seven years of progressive development of the disease. The manifestations began in the lower extremities and gradually extended to the upper. The facial muscles and those of the tongue are affected to such a degree as to make the patient's speech difficult and almost unintelligible. The extreme muscular activity seems to be due to sustained tonic spasms in a large number of muscle groups, many of which are not pertinent to the particular motor act. These spasms produce distortions of the body with marked deformity of motion.

At the usual cinematographic rate of reproduction, the patient bears a strong resemblance in her gait, attitude and posture to the brother and sister. There is a similar flexor fixation at the knees with an equinus fixation of the feet when the patient stands. In locomotion the right heel fails to reach the floor. The typical pronation position of the forearms is emphasized.

In the slow motion pictures, analysis disclosed typical hyperkinetic and hyperstatic disturbances. The marked overflow of innervation is apparent in nearly every group of muscles in the body, producing needless and often untimely postures as well as movements wholly unnecessary for the acts performed.

EPIDEMIC ENCEPHALITIS

(Film running time: 19 minutes)

Each case presents some particular feature of the disease giving it diagnostic value and scientific interest. These graphic visualizations present sequential histories, in most cases, over a period of years of observation. Some of the patients show the earliest manifestations of the developing clinical pathology.

Case 1—Case showing champing (chewing) movements following in a few months a mild attack of acute encephalitis. One year after this picture was taken there developed a Parkinsonian posture and a psychosis with delusional trends; the patient committed suicide some months later.

One sees constant champing movements of the lower jaw and a masked facies. These champing movements are present with the mouth open or closed. They are slow, approximately 40 per minute, regular and rhythmical. The persisting paresis of the internal rectus muscle of the left eye is a sequela of the acute illness.

Case 2—Patient showing another type of champing movements. Acute encephalitis in 1920 with apparently complete recovery. Two years later the present symptoms appeared.

Patient stands in rigid posture with arms and legs semi-flexed and trunk bowed slightly forward; typical posture of paralysis agitans with Parkinsonian facies and oiliness of the skin. Champing movements in this case are apparently due to automatic physiological response to the unusual condition, in this case, of deficiency of salivary secretion. (This patient did not show the excessive salivation usually seen.) Champing movements cease both when the mouth is open and also upon voluntary closure of the eyes. The gait shows loss of associated movements in the upper extremities.

Case 3—Film was taken shortly after acute encephalitis. There is rigidity of facial musculature, with changes in facial contour suggesting the process of rapid aging since onset of the illness.

Patient shows anxious, fixed expression with the tremors limited to tongue and lips.

Case 4—As in the preceding case, physical signs of rapid aging followed the acute attack; here, too, are seen tremors of tongue and lips and rigidity of facial muscles.

Case 5—Patient shows Parkinsonian syndrome and some thalamic symptoms. He has an alert, though fixed expression, and there are sudden outbursts of spontaneous and automatic smiling and laughter.

Case 6—Acute illness in February 1920. Very severe extensive involvement of the cerebro-spinal system with rapid progression to the condition presented here, July 1922.

Before the acute illness, patient was a professional toe dancer. The almost universal involvement of the central nervous system, as shown in this case, is rarely seen. Due to bilateral involvement of the fifth nerve nucleus during her acute illness, she developed a corneal anesthesia with subsequent neuroparalytic keratitis and gradual loss of vision. There is also involvement of lower motor-neuron systems. There were trophic ulcerations of the body; one large trophic ulcer involved the right hip. The patient's head is tilted to the left and all bodily movements are restricted or distorted, indicative of extensive pathology. The posture suggests a dystonic fragment, and one sees fragmentary spontaneous movements of both lower extremities. There is a slight extension movement of the right leg and flexion and extension movement at the left hip and knee; in form and design these appear to be a type of compulsion movements. This patient suffered from almost continuous intense headache.

Case 7—Acute encephalitis in 1918. The first scene taken three years later shows bilateral dystonic postural design with tremors.

The same patient shown one year later presents tremors and contractures and prolonged paroxysms of turning and fixation of the head and eyes, in extreme lateral position (encephalo-oculogyric crises). At this time she also experienced inversion of the day and night periods; the fixed postures present throughout the day disappeared completely at night and with this change the lethargy of the daytime was replaced by mental alertness. Her nocturnal activities included constant wandering about the wards and frequent visits to the cupboard. An occasional spontaneous smile and laughter of encephalitic design can be seen momentarily in the picture.

Patient is presented on the screen in her typical posture of the daytime. Tremors are present in all extremities, but the rate and rhythm seen in the upper differ from those of the lower. A typical encephalo-oculo-gyric crisis is shown; observe spasmodic contraction of the right sternocleidomastoid muscle, turning the head to the left and fixing it in that position; simultaneously the eyes are rotated and fixed in the left lateral position. These periodic seizures lasted, as a rule, thirteen hours. Observe Magnus de Kleijn design of posture—flexion of the right arm and extension of the left with the head turned to the left. This postural entity appeared as spontaneously assumed irregular periodic seizures.

Case 8—Outstanding in this picture are the so-called "intention tremors" (dyssynergia, as seen in multiple sclerosis).

In this patient, tremors of wide amplitude of the head, face, tongue, trunk and extremities are seen to become greatly accentuated during active movements. Finger to finger and finger to nose tests show almost total disintegration of coordinated movements; observe disorganization of timing and rhythm of speech musculature in attempted articulation.

Case 9—Acute encephalitis showing myoclonic movements.

This case shows myoclonic movements of the abdominal muscles and those of the thigh causing external rotation of the entire left lower extremity. These movements are sudden, tic-like, spontaneous and rapidly recurrent.

Case 10—The studies of this patient were also made during the early period of the acute attack. Massive myoclonic movements in the lower extremities are shown. These movements were preceded by radicular pains in the areas involved.

The scenes demonstrate the voluminous involvement of quadriceps, hamstring and gluteal groups of muscles.

Same patient *two years* later—only occasional attacks of muscular twitchings in the lower extremities remain.

Same patient *three years* after acute illness—apparently there is complete recovery and all muscular movements are under perfect voluntary control; no involuntary or abnormal movments are seen. This patient is shown in various attitudes to demonstrate the normal activity and voluntary control in the motor system.

The last two cases were first filmed at the height of the acute attack; in both, the general constitutional symptoms were severe.

Case 11—Boy age 14. Acute illness in 1920 was followed by severe general choreiform movements. The later development of the Parkinsonian syndrome is now shown.

We now see a typical Parkinsonian facial expression with its characteristic elements of fixation, immobility and alertness. The gait and posture show latero-, pro, and retropulsion, characteristic rigidity and wax-like configuration of trunk and body segments with loss of normal associated movements. When seated, during testing of muscle tone in the upper extremity (for cogwheel phenomenon), observe that patient falls into momentary somnolence, common to acute and subacute phases of epidemic encephalitis.

Cases 12 and 13—These two cases show extreme flexion posture with forward falling. Note the maintenance of increased muscle tone in the first patient, in spite of the dissolution of posture. This increased tone is not as evident in the second case. In the second case note also the peculiar smile so typical in design of the post-encephalitic subject. One is reminded of a cataplectic seizure.

Case 14—10 years of age, presented shortly after his acute illness, shows compulsive type of involuntary flexion movements of the lower extremities, of greater amplitude on the right. These motor phenomena are spontaneous and apparently repetitive in design. There is a tendency towards adduction of the right lower extremity with the extension movement and slight rotation of the body to the left. There are tremors of both upper extremities, greater on the right than on the left. One also observes compulsive opening and closing of the mouth—a sucking design—and spontaneous flexion and adduction of the left upper extremity. Observe that when attempts are made to induce and help the patient walk, there is a breaking up of the entire pattern of walking with spontaneous flexion movements of both lower extremities at the thighs. As shown, these gross movements can be induced by passive flexion of the head on the body when the patient lies supine. These movements are of especial interest, demonstrating, as they do in the human, the same design of "progression movements" as experimentally produced by Graham-Brown in lower animals.

Case 15—Acute encephalitis in 1920. One year later the present clinical picture developed and up to March 1926, at which time these pictures were taken, the condition remained unchanged.

There is involuntary opening of the mouth which is impeded or relieved when the patient speaks, chews or swallows. Mimetic stimulation (laughing) at times stops the involuntary oral movements. In walking there is a loss of associated movements of the upper extremities and the mouth is held open. The gait is slow, deliberate and the patient tends to drag the left leg but there is no evidence of pyramdial system involvement.

Case 16—Among other features of interest this case shows unilateral tic-like movements of all segments of the body, in design suggestive of the preagonal movements seen in the final moments of dissolution in the human. Note the youth of the patient as one sees her here, and compare these early scenes with the later ones, showing the patient appearing many years older, in a very brief period of time.

There is partial suppression of normal associated movements of the left upper extremity in walking. When seated note the "hiking" of the left leg in a tic-like manner and also spontaneous extension of the left big toe, and synchronously a similar type of movement of the left upper extremity; these movements are all involuntary and spontaneous. We have here a combination of pyramidal and extrapyramidal signs. Associated with these abnormal movements is a slight backward and rotary movement of the head to the right. The left supra-nuclear facial paresis is a residual of the acute stage of her illness. One year later a profound change in posture, general appearance and clinical signs developed. The abnormal movements have ceased and the clinical picture is replaced by a typical Parkinsonian syndrome; within the short period of 12 months the patient appears to have rapidly aged, showing, among other signs, an increase in adiposity with marked transition in facial expression and bodily posture and contour. The influence of tone upon the determination of posture remains a problem in neurophysiology; the case presented tends to show that design of posture (as in Parkinsonism) is determined by a mechanism quite independent of the degree of tone, for in this case the examiner demonstrates an absence of hypertonia of the muscle groups concerned in maintenance of posture in the upper extremities.

Case 17—Acute illness (epidemic form) in 1920. The changes, as shown in her present condition, began two years later. There developed a marked and striking change in facial contour and expression. Signs of profound changes in endocrine function appeared.

The case illustrates the striking physical transformation which sometimes follows the acute attack. Before her acute illness this woman was an active, intelligent and physically attractive person. One now sees marked hirsutism and typical Parkinsonian posture. The hair of her head, formerly of fine texture, has become bristle-like and wiry, the skin rough and oily. During moments of emotional stress, she suddenly perspires so excessively that she appears as though having just emerged from a bath. Vegetative centers were involved in the pathological process.

Case 18—A young girl of 16 years of age with chronic epidemic encephalitis gouges out both eyes while under observation in a general hospital. During the preceding two years she had pulled out all but seven of her teeth.

The history up to February 1923 showed a normal background. About this time she suffered an acute attack of influenza followed a year later by a left hemi-parkinson motor syndrome.

During her first year at High School a lack of concentration and sustained effort were reported. "Spasms of the eye lids" and changes in personality made her a behavior problem at home. When she was confronted with the results of her destructive conduct she admitted her misdoings and said she could not help it; at times she showed remorse and would spontaneously reiterate "Why do I do it; why do I do it; I can't help it". Her tantrums would occasionally be followed by a brief period of somnolence.

The patient was admitted to Morrisania Hospital on July 30th, 1931 because of slight swelling and redness of the right eye caused by the patient rubbing her eye during the day. On entering the Hospital the eye was given local treatments. The patient was quiet and apparently slept until early morning. A short time later a nurse, called suddenly to the patient's room, found the girl lying quietly in bed holding her avulsed right eye in her hand. The patient said the eye had spontaneously fallen out while she was sleeping. The patient replied in an intelligent and unhesitating manner to all questions put to her. She was not at all perturbed and did not complain of pain or discomfort. Her actions were quite normal except for a seeming indifference toward the incident. About one and a half hours later the patient suddenly shouted and the nurse who went to her bedside was told by the patient that the left eye had "popped" out. The eye was found in the bed at the patient's left side; there was only slight bleeding from the orbital cavity. The patient lay quietly, without evidence of emotion; she was well oriented and her remote memory was good. She insisted that she did not recall the details of that particular period when her eyes "popped" out. There was no intellectual defect. Her responses to sensory examination were normal; indeed, she was quite sensitive to pin-prick in all areas. The only physical neurological defect was the old left extrapyramidal hemiplegia. The eyes were enucleated, practically intact. The eye muscles were torn at the tendons in both eyes; the optic nerves were also avulsed; the right nerve attached to the eyeball was an inch long and the left nearly two inches.

In October 1931 she was transferred to the Neuropsychiatric service of the Montefiore Hospital. During the first two weeks of her stay there she attempted many times to injure herself; she declared a force within herself "made her do these things"; she was restrained and carefully watched. She was taught to read by the Braille system while at the Hospital and was an apt pupil.

As seen in the film, she is undernourished, edentulous and with empty orbits. Mentally she was cooperative in ward routine although displaying some irritability and emotional instability. There were no spontaneous productions and her stream of thought was normal; she had no delusions or hallucinations and no bizarre ideas. Her affective reactions were apparently adequate and there was no dissociation of affect. She showed a real sense of humor and was much interested in what was going on; she was alert to any changes in her immediate environment and, as might be expected, she had an exceedingly keen sense of hearing; indeed, she was able to recognize and differentiate individuals immediately upon hearing the voice. Her reaction to discussion of her self-mutilation would be that of momentary depression and she avoided any reference to the episodes. She invariably stated that she did not remember anything of the period during which her eyes, as she expressed it, "popped out".

In July 1932 she began to show some mild mental symptoms of paranoidal color. She was admitted to the Manhattan State Hospital April 16, 1937. She gradually became exceedingly obese and apathetic. On one occasion, apparently under an obsessional compulsion, she infected her right index finger, the one used for Braille, by rubbing it on the metal part of the mattress during the night. The finger was later amputated. She died July 23, 1940; the diagnosis, post-mortem, was bronchopneumonia; postencephalitic exhaustive psychosis.*

Case 19—A female patient showing, in the presence of an extrapyramidal hemiplegia, an unusual posture of the right hand with a dystonic attitude of the right lower extremity.

She presents a typical picture of Parkinsonism. The right hand is closed with strongly flexed fingers. Both arms are flexed at the elbow, the left more than the right. The right lower extremity is partially flexed at the knee and the foot assumes the dystonic posture of extension and inversion. In walking, the posture becomes more emphasized, so that on the right foot she walks on the toes.

This case illustrates the typical fixed dystonic posture and wax-like rigidity of encephalitic origin.

---

*A detailed account of this case and review of the literature was published by S. P. Goodhart, M.D. and Nathan Savitsky, M.D.; "Self-mutilation in Chronic Encephalitis", American Journal of the Medical Sciences, May 1933; Number 5.

Case 20—Patient is a 10-year-old boy whose acute illness occurred in 1922, at which time he showed bulbar involvement. His present motor seizures followed one month later.

He shows spontaneous forced extension of the head and synchronous opening of the mouth with extension and pronation of the arms, an attitude suggesting the decerebrate type of rigidity. Pictures taken six weeks later show some changes with temporary improvement; however, variability in clinical signs in such cases is not unusual; the patient is here seen walking with an almost normal gait. This apparent synchronization of arm and leg movement is due to instruction and an effort at reeducation.

Pictures taken about three years later (March 1926) visualize the beginning of what ultimately became a classical syndrome of Parkinsonism with its posture, facies and gait.

Case 21—A man 37 years old, showing an unusual type of rhythmical movement of his right arm and leg with typical Parkinsonian tremor of the left arm and leg.

In this case we see the residua of acute encephalitis. It is of interest to note that the design of these movements is strikingly suggestive of the so-called "Flügelschlagen" (wing-beating) movements seen in hepatolenticular degeneration. (The Flügelschlagen movements are classically demonstrated in another group of pictures of patients, showing hepatolenticular degeneration).

Case 22—This patient demonstrates a classical picture of posture and gait with pro- and retropulsion in Parkinsonism. Festination, with retropulsion, is seen in the final pictures.

FRIEDREICH'S HEREDITARY ATAXIA

(Film running time: 10 minutes)

Friedreich's Hereditary Ataxia is a heredo-degenerative spino-cerebellar disease. It presents a clinical syndrome, expressive of degenerative nature, of the dorsal and lateral half of the spinal cord and of the cerebellum and, not infrequently, the presence of developmental anomalies of the nervous system and other structures. The onset is usually at puberty (between the 7th and 15th year of life); the first symptoms occasionally appear later. The syndrome consists of ataxia both of the cerebellar and posterior column type; the extremities and the trunk may be involved. The degree of ataxia varies with the progress of the disease. There is also nystagmus, kyphoscoliosis and characteristic deformity or rather contour of the feet; the latter suggests a dystonic design and is known as "Friedreich's foot"; (a very high arch of peculiar contour and a relative short foot with tendency to chronic extensor position of the big toe) it shows a definite pes cavus. The hand likewise shows characteristic structural contour known as manus cavus. There is some degree of muscular weakness with hypotonia.

The sensory changes involve the modalities of vibration, joint-muscle-tendon sense (position), stereognosis, two-point discrimination and tactile in mild degree.

The deep reflexes of the lower extremities are absent; plantar stimulation elicits extensor response (Babinski). These two signs are due to involvement of posterior columns and pyramidal tracts. There may be optic atrophy and not infrequently, there is general undersized skeletal structure.

The pathology shows a primary degeneration of the pyramidal, spino-cerebellar and dorsal column tracts in the spinal cord, often with degenerative disease in the cerebellum; the latter has frequently been found atrophic, the ganglion cells reduced in number and the Purkinje cells not infrequently entirely absent. Two related entities are recognized: the spinal hereditary ataxia (Friedreich) and the cerebellar hereditary ataxia (Pierre Marie). Fragments of each type may be occasionally observed in the same patient.

A group of four patients is presented showing classical signs of this disease; these include two brothers in one family and two sisters in another. Some observers have also placed in this group rather rare forms of localized pathology probably allied to this disease; these are Marie's cerebellar heredo-ataxia and primary progressive cerebellar degeneration (of Holmes).

Case 1—24 years of age. The patient's gait shows disturbance in equilibrium; this defect is of the cerebellar type of motor incoordination. The positive Romberg test and the absence of deep reflexes indicate involvement of the posterior columns also. Pathology in the pyramidal tracts is shown by the extensor plantar responses (Babinski sign).

Case 2—22 years of age, brother of preceding patient showing much more advanced condition. The gait here is definitely of cerebellar (dyssynergic) origin with breaking up of intersegmental coordination. This case shows both pes cavus and manus cavus, also absence of the patellar and ankle reflexes with bilateral extensor plantar responses. The generalized cerebellar ataxia and hypotonia, involving also the trunk, is further demonstrated when the patient, seated, endeavors to arise.

Case 3—23 years of age, the older of two sisters, demonstrates a marked cerebellar gait; she cannot walk without assistance. Typical so-called "Friedreich's foot" is shown—pes cavus and permanent hyperextension of the big toe with flexion of its distal phalanx. Further neurological signs demonstrated in this patient are bilateral pyramidal tract involvement—extensor plantar responses; posterior column pathology—absent patellar reflexes and disturbances of joint-muscle-tendon sense as shown in the finger to finger test with the patient's eyes closed.

Case 4—21 years of age, sister of the preceding patient; her condition is more advanced. The gait is characteristic of involvement of both the cerebellum and posterior columns. Evidence of the defect in function of the posterior columns is indicated by the constant use of vision in maintaining equilibrium in walking and in the efforts at correction of ataxia while performing the finger to finger and finger to nose tests. The dyssynergia as shown by the incoordination between agonist and antagonist groups of muscles, in performing the latter tests, is of cerebellar character.

LITTLE'S DISEASE AND DOUBLE ATHETOSIS

To convey an idea of the clinical varieties of what is called Little's Disease, the following may be given as the most common designations: Little's disease; cerebral diplegia; infantile cerebral hemiplegia; cerebellar diplegia; hereditary spastic paraplegia or diplegia. Thus we see Little's disease is not a definite disease entity but rather appears as any one of several syndromes; pyramidal, extra-pyramidal, or a combination of these may be the nervous structures involved with corresponding clinical picture. The condition has its origin in natal or prenatal life. The causes are numerous, the more common being trauma, infection or vascular lesions. Convulsive seizures are not uncommon. Involvement of supranuclear structures may give pseudobulbar symptoms—defect in speech and swallowing. The mentality may be normal or show mild or profound defect from normalcy to idiocy. The pathology, naturally, is a varied one both in nature and location. There may be scattered small cicatricial lesions or extensive extravasations, effusions of blood, punctate hemorrhages, internal and external hydrocephalus and porencephaly. Any of these may be the source or result of pathological change within the cranium. A congenital aplasia is doubtless the cause in some cases.

Double athetosis is really a type of Little's disease and affects both halves of the body segments. The classic type of dyskinesia is that seen in the most distal parts of the extremities; other segments may be involved—face and tongue. The design is that of so-called mobile spasm, constant alternate hyperextension and flexion; the design of movement in fingers and toes is vermicular and may be compared to that of the tentacles of the octopus. The idiopathic form—Athetosis Doublé—bilateral congenital athetosis, is really a syndrome sui generis. Because of involvement of the tongue and face, constant grimacing, disturbance in articulation and head and neck movements accompany those of the extremities. The cortico-spinal pathways are involved with pathology in the corpus striatum.

A group of cases is presented showing various forms of dyskinesias of congenital origin. The abnormal movements are predominantly of extrapyramidal type. The diffuse pathology of these cases makes exact classification inadvisable. There may be fragmentary choreiform, athetotic and dystonic elements. An encephalographic study of these cases is presented in another film.

LITTLE'S DISEASE AND DOUBLE ATHETOSIS

Case 1—32 years of age. The impressive feature in this case is the extensive athetosis in the upper and, to a lesser degree, in the lower extremities. Choreiform elements and facial grimacing are also present. As part of this congenital picture, there is marked intellectual retardation.

Case 2—30 years of age, congenital spastic triplegia. The left upper extremity is unaffected. The bilateral spasticity and gait are indicative of involvement of the pyramidal system.

Case 3—37 years of age. Patient shown at 22, 37 and 44 years of age, respectively. Seated, extensive classical athetotic movements in all peripheral segments are seen. These movements, including facial grimacing congenital in origin, are still present, as demonstrated in the pictures taken fifteen and twenty years later. The dyskinesias include sudden spontaneous, irregular movements in the extremities. These are extrapyramidal in character; there is macroglossia with sialorrhoea. Speech is explosive and dysarthric in type. There is only a moderate degree of mental retardation. The athetotic movements are shown also in slow motion.

Case 4—21 years of age, shows essentially the same design of movements as seen in the preceding patients. Dystonic features are observed in the lower extremities. There is no mental deterioration; the laughter is spontaneous and automatic.

Case 5—15 years of age, also illustrates the form of movement seen in extrapyramidal entities of congenital origin.

Case 6—9 years of age. A marked feature in this case is the hyper- and hypotonicity giving dystonic character to the movements of the lower extremities. Athetotic and choreiform elements are also present.

PROGRESSIVE MUSCULAR ATROPHIES PSEUDOHYPERTROPHIES AND ALLIED CONDITIONS

(Film running time: 15 minutes)

Pathological conditions associated with generalized muscular atrophy are numerous. One group of cases presented will demonstrate both muscle atrophy and pseudohypertrophy, primarily due, as far as we know, to a pathology within the muscle substance (dystrophies or primary myopathies).

Perhaps the term abiotrophy (Gowers), suggesting inherent defect in embryological development or biological deficiency, best explains what, at present, is known of the fundamental pathogenesis.

The term *progressive muscular atrophy* is used for another group in which the pathology is limited to the anterior horn cells of the spinal cord.

A third series of patient demonstrates conditions in which muscular atrophy is a conspicuous but not the only element in the syndrome.

PROGRESSIVE MUSCULAR ATROPHY

A chronic progressive degenerative disease of the anterior horn cells; clinical manifestations are limited to the lower motor neuron syndrome. The acral musculature is primarily involved and only later axio-appendicular groups.

Two general types are recognized; pathology is the same in both and division is based upon the initial localization. The condition may remain stationary or progress over a period of years. The clinical picture includes progressive weakness in the affected muscles in which fibrillary twitchings appear early or later; diminution, then loss of deep tendon reflexes with muscle atrophy. Electrical changes are present and progress to reaction of degeneration as the anterior horn cell degeneration advances. The pathological process in the Aran-Duchenne type, confined to the anterior horn cells, causes no sensory changes.

1. *Aran-Duchenne Type*—The first signs usually appear as weakness and wasting in the small muscles of the hands; the process extends upwards to involve forearms, arms and shoulders corresponding to the controlling cells of the cervico-brachial spinal cord area; the involvement is more or less symmetrical.

2. *Charcot-Marie Tooth Type* (also called peroneal type of neuritic atrophy—Heredo-degenerative; begins in extensors of the feet, progressing slowly upward to legs, thighs and pelvis; may soon involve upper extremities beginning in acral parts. The pathology of the anterior horn cells, may be accompanied by peripheral sensory nerve changes clinically shown as "so-called glove and stocking design"; steppage gait, due to foot-drop, is an early sign; pes equinus and club foot are often part of the picture.

PROGRESSIVE MUSCULAR DYSTROPHY

A chronic progressive wasting of skeletal musculature, frequently associated with pseudo-hypertrophy. The term "pseudo" is applied because the hypertrophy is not a true physiological enlargement. The muscles themselves are the primary seat of the pathology; there is loss of cross and later longitudinal striations, splitting of fibers and replacement of muscle fibres by connective tissue and fat; in the pseudo-hypertrophic muscles there is deposition of fat within the layers. So far as is known there is no involvement of the central or peripheral nervous system. Evidence of endocrine dysfunction may be an incidental finding or perhaps an etiological factor. The muscles showing pseudo-hypertrophy are always of the same group—deltoids and triceps in the upper and glutei and gastrocnemii in the lower extremities. The age of onset is usually between five and ten years; occasionally after puberty and more rarely in adult life (3rd decade). The disease is heredo-familiar and transmitted through the mother. The muscular dystrophies have been divided into groups with reference to the particular muscle groups involved. The fundamental pathology, so far as is now known, limited to changes within the muscle tissue, is the same in all. The division into types is of clinical interest only. The classification is rather arbitrary, the groups not sharply defined, often merging into each other.

1. An atrophic group without pseudo-hypertrophy.

2. A pseudo-hypertrophic group; in this, specious enlargement of certain muscles is an outstanding feature. (1) and (2) as a rule show first signs of involvement in early childhood and affect males predominantly. The originally pseudo-hypertrophic types often begin at about the 8th or 9th year, the purely atrophic at about the 3rd. The muscles first involved in (1) and (2) are those about the pelvic girdle and thighs.

3. Juvenile, scapulo-humeral type (Erb).

4. Infantile, facio-scapulo-humeral type (Landouzy-Dejerine), usually begins in infantile years. Later the weakness of facial musculature causes the so-called "myopathic facies" appearance—a fixed expressionless, immobile form of facial contour with a protruding upper lip (bouch de tapir).

PROGRESSIVE MUSCULAR DYSTROPHY

The clinical features of the dystrophies depend upon the loss of mechanical support of the muscles. Hence, when the shoulder and scapulohumeral groups are affected, there result so-called "wing" scapulae and "loose" shoulders; the scapulae stand out like wings when the arms are raised or are outstretched in front. When attempt is made by the examiner to raise the patient by the examiner placing the latter's hands in the patient's axillae, the shoulders cannot be fixed in position. With involvement of the pelvic group the patient walks with a "waddling" gait and the weakness of trunk muscles causes a lordosis and abdominal protrusion. In the early period of the affection, a pathognomonic series of postures is observed when the patient, lying on his back and then rising to the upright standing position, appears to "climb up" upon himself. Electrical changes of quantitative character are found; deep reflexes are diminished or disappear as the loss of muscle tissue advances.

Three illustrative groups of cases are shown here in which the distinctive feature is involvement of the body musculature. The first group is that of progressive muscular atrophies; the second, progressive muscular dystrophies; the third, conditions allied to the first two groups. The first demonstrates the Aran-Duchenne and Charcot-Marie-Tooth types of progressive muscular atrophy; the second, classical clinical pictures of the various types of progressive muscular dystrophy; the third, a series of cases of amyotonia congenita, myotonia congenita, myotonia atrophica, myasthenia gravis, syringomyelia, syringobulbia and amyotrophic lateral sclerosis.

Case 1—Male patient about 25 years of age, showing Aran-Duchenne type of progressive muscular atrophy.

This picture shows bilateral involvement of the small muscles of the hands and the muscles of the forearms. Although the atrophy is in general symmetrical, at present it is somewhat greater on the right. There is beginning atrophy of the muscles of the shoulder girdle; observe the sudden drop of both scapulae due to atrophy and weakness of their muscular attachments. The lower extremities are, as yet, not affected. As the pathology in this disease is limited to anterior horn cells, there are no sensory disturbances. The atrophy begins, as a rule, in the peripheral, acral groups.

Case 2—This is a male patient, 18 years of age, showing Charcot-Marie-Tooth type (also called peroneal type) of progressive muscular atrophy.

The illness began in the first decade of life, involving the peronei and extensor muscles of the feet, later the muscles of the upper extremities.

All modalities of sensation were mildly involved, in somewhat greater degree in the lower extremities.

Four cases of muscular dystrophy follow, showing various phases of the illness from incipient to profound involvement.

Case 3—The first patient is a boy, six years of age. The initial sign was a slight uncertainty of gait with a tendency to fall occasionally, and at times use his arms in an attempt to maintain balance; a slight but definite lordosis is seen. Although the gastrocnemius group of muscles in the leg is usually involved early, in this case the anterior tibial group is shown first affected—the patient can stand on his toes but not on his heels. The characteristic attitudes in rising, seen in the muscular dystrophies, are observed when the patient tries to arise from a supine position on the floor to the erect posture; he rises by "climbing up" upon himself.

Cases 4 and 5—Two patients presented show more advanced stages of the disease. The fact that they are brothers emphasizes the familial nature of the illness. There is marked "winging" of the scapulae, lordosis due to weakness and atrophy of the trunkal muscles, and pseudo-hypertrophy of the calf muscles more pronounced in the older boy. Note the characteristic "waddling" gait. These patients illustrate the technique used in the more advanced stages in an effort to arise from the sitting position; in bending the legs at the knees and hips, observe how they lean forward first and assume a quadruped position, then, as the knees are bent, the body suddenly collapses, to be supported as though the knees were hinges; this is largely due to the atrophic state of the quadriceps femoris group of muscles. In cases of progressive muscular dystrophy, the axio-appendicular groups of muscles are first involved, quite in contrast to the initial involvement, in progressive spinal muscular atrophy in which the distal muscle groups are first affected. In spite of the apparent enlargement (pseudo-hypertrophy) of certain of the muscles, the weakness is no less pronounced than in the atrophic groups; the pathology is a pseudo- not a physiological hypertrophy.

Case 6—This patient shows a lesser degree of muscular involvement with no hypertrophy.

Case 7—In his first pictures this patient shows the typical waddling gait, but no hypertrophy. In his effort to arise from the floor he shows the typical attitudes.

Pictures taken three years later show a marked change in the clinical

ALLIED CONDITIONS

signs. We see here the development of a pseudo-hypertrophy of both calves, more pronounced on the left. There has been an extensive deposit of fat uniformly distributed throughout the body; the adiposity as frequently seen in these cases may be related to endocrine dysfunction; further evidence of endocrine involvement is the pronounced development of hirsuties. This classical picture embodies all the important features of the clinical entity, namely: pseudo-hypertrophies, "winging" scapulae, lordosis, generalized loss of muscle power, adiposity, "waddling" gait and characteristic posture in arising, in advanced cases.

Case 8—Another case showing "loose shoulders" as a result of a loss of power in the shoulder groups of muscles.

Case 9—A case advanced to such an extent as to leave the patient bedridden. This patient is one of a group selected as illustrative of the marked endocrine changes which may accompany or, perhaps, stand in some etiological relationship to the pathology of this disease. The limitation of the patient's muscle function is shown by the few movements still possible, as demonstrated in the last pictures. An unusual finding in this case was the specific pathological change in the nonstriated cardiac muscle as disclosed by autopsy studies.

ALLIED CONDITIONS

1. *Amyotonia Congenita* (Oppenheim's Disease)—The term congenital muscular atonia has also been applied. It is a congenital pathological condition showing first signs usually between the sixth and twelfth month of life, although cases are reported in which the syndrome first appeared at a later period. There is not infrequently marked improvement and the prognosis, as to life, is fairly good; recovery, if it does occur, is rarely complete.

The syndrome presents a flaccid paralysis affecting all or only some segments of the body, absent deep reflexes, quantitatively reduced electrical responses. Mentality, speech, sensation, and sphincters are unaffected. Other congenital anomalies are occasionally found. A striking feature, resulting from the flaccid state of the muscles and the loose joints, is the bizarre positions into which arms and legs can be placed. The contortions are extreme; the patient, at times, can seemingly be "tied into knots". The seat and nature of the pathology are not definitely determined. The disease may be an expression of prenatal changes, or defective development of anterior horn cells. The ventral roots are thin, not fully developed, and deficient in myelin.

2. *Myotonia Congenita* (Thomsen's Disease) —A familial congenital

disease usually beginning in childhood, but sometimes first becoming evident at puberty or later. Patients are frequently of excellent physique and unusual size, the seeming hypertrophy sometimes apparent in upper or lower extremities or in all. The obtrusive sign is defective motility by reason of tonic spasm or what is called myotonus. There is a heightened contractility of the voluntary musculature with a slowing of voluntary relaxation, a failure of muscles to relax promptly—the myotonic reaction. After repeated slow, voluntary attempts at relaxation and contraction the muscles finally "loosen-up"—the tonic spasm ceases, enabling the normal movement to be completed. The finer changes in muscles strongly suggest a relationship in pathology between myotonia congenita and muscular dystrophy; increased sarcoplasm and some increase in sarcolemmal cells are found and implication of the myoneural junction is probable. The influence of quinine in relieving the condition and of prostigmin in intensifying the symptoms is significant perhaps of physiological or biochemical implication.

3. *Myotonia Atrophica* (Dystrophia Myotonica)—A heredo-degenerative disease; onset between the 20th and 30th year; characterized by so-called "hatchet-facies" due to atrophy of the masseter and temporal muscles; "pole neck" due to wasting of the sternocleidomastoid muscles; the development in early life of ocular cataracts; baldness; atrophy of testicles or ovaries; as a rule the myotonic reaction is present.

The pathology is much like that found in the muscle tissue in progressive muscular dystrophy. Victims of the disease rarely live beyond the middle life period.

4. *Myasthenia Gravis*—The clinical features of the syndrome are rapid progressive development of weakness in apparently normal voluntary muscles, power returning after a brief period of rest. The muscles affected exhaust rapidly after functioning. Wasting of muscle is sometimes observed and thus a clinical resemblance to the dystrophies is suggested; because of the frequent involvement of muscles of cranial nerve innervation, a clinical analogy to bulbar palsy symptomatology appears in some cases. No definite signs or evidence of involvement of the central, or peripheral nervous system, have been determined. Sensation remains intact. The early signs and symptoms are usually observed between the ages of 20 and 40 years. Although, as stated, predeliction is for ocular muscles and those of the face, lips, jaws, throat and neck, later nearly all of the striated muscles may be involved. Rapid exhaustion in the muscles of mastication and of deglutition during taking of food and weakness of the neck muscles may be an early sign. The voice may be quickly reduced to a whisper when muscles of the vocal cords are involved.

A peculiarity of the syndrome of exhaustion and weakness is the relation between rapidly repeated movements and onset of fatigue; the latter is often greatest at the close of the day. Ptosis of the upper lids is observed in some cases only late in the day and a night's rest usually favorably influences the patient's morning condition. Naturally, in some cases, walking and repeated use of a group of trunk or segmental muscles cause complete loss of power, quickly restored by an interval of rest. In nearly all cases persistent weakness and exhaustion finally occur. Diplopia due to ocular muscle involvement is often an early symptom.

The pathology is really undetermined; biochemical changes are suspected—disturbance in acetycholine catabolism (rapid breaking up of acetycholine by its specific estorase) with disturbance in the transmission of impulses past the myoneural junction; biopsy of affected muscles shows the presence of "lymphorrhagia", an infiltration of muscles with round cells; a persistent thymus gland is sometimes found.

The favorable influence of prostigmin in Myasthenia Gravis is most striking, usually enabling the patient to continue muscle function with far greater efficiency.

The prognosis is uncertain. Recovery has been reported. Patients may succumb in a few years; others last for many years with periods of improvement and of exacerbation.

5. *Syringomyelia*—A chronic progressive disease characterized by loss of appreciation of pain and temperature stimuli with preservation of touch; muscle atrophies and fibrillations, and often signs due to involvement of anterior horns, pyramidal tracts and posterior columns with corresponding column signs. The initial characteristic feature is the sensory dissociation (involvement of pain and temperature tracts only). The signs vary in site and extent of the pathological process. If the cervical sympathetic area (7th and 8th segments) is involved, a "Horner's Syndrome" results (contracted pupil, forearm muscle atrophy).

The disease is due to a degenerative process, secondary to congenital dysgenesis or a necrosis of cord tissue, from any cause, usually with cavity formation (syrinx), which may or may not be connected with the central canal of the cord. The pathological process may extend in various directions within the cord destroying contiguous structures. Instead of cavity formation there may be a solid mass consisting of glial tissue—central gliosis. The syrinx may be associated with the spinal cord tumor mass or with a hypertrophic pacchymeningitis. The symptoms and signs can appear at any age although usually in the second or third decade.

6. *Syringobulbia*—When the syringomyelic process extends upward involving the medulla or pons or both, cranial nerve nuclei and funi-

cular systems in this area become the seat of the pathology with resulting signs and symptoms.

AMYOTROPHIC LATERAL SCLEROSIS

A disease classified as degenerative, commonly observed in the middle period of life, 30 to 55, occasionally earlier. The classical syndrome first described by Charcot includes weakness and atrophy in the upper extremities, spasticity and pyramidal tract signs in the lower. The name implies involvement of both upper and lower motor neurons—pyramidal tracts and anterior horn cells. Clinically two definite forms or rather motor syndromes are observed, differing only in their localization and usually merging; the pathological process may first attack bulbar and pons structures or their analogous anterior horn cells and pyramidal tracts in the spinal cord. In the former, we have the clinical picture of bulbar palsy and in the other, of progressive muscular atrophy and pyramidal tract signs. A combination of these two pathological pictures is common. Since the process is usually confined to Betz cells in the motor cortex, pyramidal tracts, motor cranial nerve nuclei and anterior horn cells in the cord, sensory changes are not a part of the clinical picture; fibrillations of affected muscles are often among early signs. The early electrical reactions, as a rule, show quantitative changes only, dependent upon the degree of atrophy. Reaction of degeneration is seen when the anterior horn cells are markedly degenerated; with dominant degeneration in the lower motor neuron, mild polar changes are found in the galvanic reaction and faradic responses continue only slightly reduced. Although sensory changes are very rarely determined, paraesthesiae and muscle cramps are occasional symptoms. With involvement of the sympathetic group in the anterior horn in the cervical region, vasomotor and ocular signs (Horner syndrome) may also be seen. Mental symptoms, either in the emotional or intellectual sphere, are not infrequent. Thus the pathology can not, in all cases, be confined to the motor system and it is indeed subject to many variations both in character and localization. The classical picture, however, is as described above.

While the syndrome in its many variations has been ascribed to different causes, its origin and etiology are undetermined. Fatal termination occurs usually in from three to five years.

A group of patients demonstrating syndromes allied, in their motor phase, to muscular dystrophies and atrophies. This group is comprised of the following entities: amyotonia congenita *(Oppenheim's disease),* myotonia congenita *(Thomsen's disease) ,* myotonia atrophica, myasthenia gravis, syringomyelia, syringobulbia, amyotrophic lateral sclerosis.

Case 1—A female child, four and one half years of age, who has never been able to stand or walk and is barely able to sit up because of marked hypotonicity and weakness of the muscles. These passively produced attitudes demonstrate the extreme hypotonicity as found in amyotonia congenita (Oppenheim's disease). Observe the marked degree to which hyperextension and hyperflexion can be induced.

Case 2—This case of myotonia congenita (Thomsen's disease) demonstrates the classical feature—inability of the patient to spontaneously relax a voluntarily contracted group of muscles. Thus, closing his eyes, he is unable to open them for a few seconds; illustrative of the same phenomenon is his inability to open his closed hands or to spontaneously open his closed mouth (observe contraction of platysma muscle). The same phenomenon is seen in other muscle groups; it is due to a sustained myotonic contraction of the initiating group of muscles. Another feature of the disease is the myotonic contraction when the muscle bundle is struck; observe this in the tongue and thenar eminence when they are mechanically stimulated by a blow and you then see the cramp-like muscular contraction. With the relaxation of muscle reaction, note the facility with which the voluntary movement can then be continuously repeated.

Case 3—A case of myotonia atrophica is shown in a woman aged 42, whose brother was afflicted with the same illness; both parents had congenital bilateral cataracts. The salient features are: "hatchet facies", the result of atrophy of the temporal and masseter muscles; "pole neck", due to atrophy of the sternocleidomastoid and trapezius muscles; ptosis of the eye-lids, caused by weakness of the levator palpebrae superioris muscles; involvement of the peroneal groups of muscles is shown on the film in patient's inability to stand on the heels; the myotonic reaction is demonstrated in the small muscles of the hands and in the tongue. The weakness of the sternocleidomastoid muscles is evidenced by the inability of the patient to overcome very slight resistance on the part of the examiner, to patient's endeavor to rotate the head laterally.

Case 4—Male patient, 49 years of age, suffering from myasthenia gravis; involvement of all voluntary groups of muscles. The pictures show patient walking back and forth for a few minutes; there results a rapidly developing onset of generalized weakness progressing to such a degree that the man soon falls to the floor; observe how laborious and increasingly difficult walking becomes for him, and the intensive effort required in his endeavor to lift his legs and propel himself forward. After a few moments of rest he becomes again able to use his muscles as well as he did in the beginning of the exercise. There is no evidence of wasting or atrophy of muscles. To further demonstrate the type and degree of weakness present, the patient, while seated in a chair, repeatedly elevates both arms from the horizontal to the extreme vertical position and in so doing shows rapidly progressing weakness, so that he is soon totally unable to elevate the arms from the horizontal position. A brief period of rest restores function.

Case 5—Another male patient demonstrating myasthenia gravis in whom the only apparent signs were involvement of the external ocular muscles and of the levator palpebrae superioris. As the patient fixes his gaze on an object moving back and forth horizontally, there is increasing fatigue of the above named muscles with gradual development of ptosis and external ophthalmoplegia. Note that as ptosis develops the patient brings into action the orbicularis oculi and frontalis muscles in an effort to keep the eyes open. Each eye is tested separately. Note again that, with rest, function returns.

Case 6—Syringomyelia, in a woman of 42, showing motor and sensory involvement of all extremities; there is characteristic sensory dissociation (touch intact, pain and temperature sensibility impaired); encroachment of the pathological process upon the anterior horn cells is evidenced by the loss of power, atrophy and fibrillations in some of the muscles, especially of the forearm. Note the peculiar characteristic contour of the hand and forearm as often seen in syringomyelia, and observe narrowing of the left palpebral fissure and myosis of the left pupil due to involvement of the sympathetic system at the level of the eighth cervical and first dorsal cord segment (Horner's Syndrome).

Case 7—A male patient, at this time 29 years of age, with syringobulbia, observed over a period of ten years. He has bulbar nuclei involvement of the nuclei of the fifth, sixth, seventh and twelfth cranial nerves with resulting motor disturbance of the muscles supplied by these nerves. The trunk and extremities participated in the characteristic sensory dissociation. The left external rectus muscle palsy is demonstrated in the patient's inability to move his left eye outward past the midline. Involvement of the nucleus of the seventh cranial nerve is evidenced by the peripheral type of facial palsy. The left half of the tongue is markedly atrophied and shows classical fibrillations. In spite of the extensive pathology the patient maintained a considerable degree of working capacity over the period of ten years of observation.

Case 8—A case of amyotrophic lateral sclerosis in a 57 year old male patient. There is involvement of the pyramidal tracts and anterior horn cells. The process extended from the cervical cord into the bulb to include the nuclei of the ninth, tenth, eleventh and twelfth cranial nerves. There is hypertonicity with exaggerated deep reflexes in some groups, ankle and patellar clonus, and pathological reflexes (upper neuron involvement), in the presence of extensive atrophy and fibrillations in other muscles (lower motor neuron). Involvement of the twelfth nerve nuclei, bilaterally, is shown by partial atrophy and inability to protrude and freely move his tongue. There is no sensory involvement.

PROGRESSIVE HEPATO-LENTICULAR DEGENERATION

(Film running time: 9 minutes)

Until Wilson, in 1912, clearly set forth the clinical and pathological findings and thus brought together a group of cases of extrapyramidal and basal ganglia pathology, progressive hepato-lenticular degeneration was unknown as an entity. The disease is familial and degenerative but not hereditary. It may appear in acute form rapidly progressive and fatal in a few months or its course may be insidious, chronic and fatal only after many years.

Pathology is found both within the brain and the liver. The cerebral findings consist chiefly of softening and degeneration of the lenticular nuclei (grossly-softening, shrinkage, cavitation) and, in a lesser degree, of the pallida. Histopathologically there is a gradual destruction of parenchyma and its replacement by glial overgrowth with degeneration and cavity formation; hepatic cirrhosis is always present and occasionally enlargement of the spleen and proliferative degeneration within the thyroid.

The clinical manifestations are largely confined to those expressive of disease of the extrapyramidal system and higher centers for intellectual function. The involuntary movments appear as tremors, and among the bizarre forms of motor manifestations are so-called "flügelschlagen", or wing-beating movements, because they are comparable in design to the flapping of wings of a bird as it flies; the amplitude of this characteristic form of movement varies. It may be confined at first to small segments, as in the fingers, or may affect all extremities; it is more often seen first in the arms. Other classical motor signs are rigidity of extrapyramidal type, dysarthria and dysphagia. In some cases symptoms, usually transient, unspecific in character, and over-emotional reactions are present and not infrequently an odd expression of the face, as the mouth remains open. Although not present in all cases, a peculiar ring on the outer surface of the cornea is a characteristic and specific finding; it appears as a greenish-brown pigment around the periphery of the cornea; a slit lamp may be required for its recognition. This pigment deposit is known as the "Kayser-Fleischer" ring.

This group of cases has its pathology in the extrapyramidal system

HEPATO-LENTICULAR DEGENERATION

and one of its distinctive features is involvement of liver structure in the form of cirrhosis. The group includes Wilson's disease, Westphal-Strumpel pseudosclerosis seen in the early decades and a group of cases of hepato-lenticular degeneration appearing in later life. Those occuring in early life belong to the heredo-degenerative diseases and are usually familial.

Case 1—24 year old woman. The striking feature in the first scenes presented is a form of involuntary compulsive movement of a distinctive design. With the upper extremities outstretched and pronated, there are extensive up-and-down vertical movements which, because of their similarity in design to the flapping of wings, have been called flugelschlagen (wing-beating) movements. Alteration in posture of the affected extremities, for example, changing to supination, causes their momentary cessation. No synergistic disturbance occurs in the finger to nose test; however, with an endeavor to maintain the approximation of finger to nose, there is a breaking up of the maintenance of this posture. The cephalic segment (head) shows the same form of movement. Another feature of the disease is that, encircling the corneal-scleral junction, there is pigment deposit known as the Kayser-Fleischer ring.

The first signs of the disease in this patient appeared at puberty. Mental changes, such as are often seen in cases of paranoid schizophrenia, were first observed when she was 26 years old and she soon required institutional care. An older brother was a victim of the same disease and likewise became psychotic.

Case 2—A 28 year old male. Before admission to Montefiore Hospital, the patient was treated for three years as a purely psychogenic case. A survey of the family history showed no other member afflicted with this disease. The type of movement seen and described in the previous case is demonstrated in this patient. The fundamental design of the dyskinsia is also seen in the lower extremities. There is, in addition, a Parksonian facies with dysarthria, as seen in pathology within the extrapyramidal system. The dysarthria is made evident in the pictures by the manifest incoordination of the muscles used in the act of articulation.

Case 3—17 years of age, was under observation at the Montefiore Hospital for twelve years. Two siblings, a sister and brother, suffered from the same syndrome. The brother died and postmortem examination revealed typical lesions of the extrapyramidal system and cirrhosis of the liver. In the patient presented here, the first signs of the disease appeared in her 13th year. It is of interest to note that, as in two other patients to be shown later, the first manifestations were suggestive of disturbance of hepatic function in the form of gastro-intestinal symptoms; liver function tests, in this patient, disclosed early impairment of hepatic activity, a condition observed in other cases we were enabled to study. In the patient presented, the classical design of "wing-beating movements" is seen and a defect in the performance of rapid alternating movements (dysdiadokokinesis) and also dyssynergia, as shown in the finger to nose test. Subsequent pictures were taken showing progress of the disease and are demonstrated on the screen.

Pictures taken five years later demonstrate the segmental limitations possible in the expression of this type of movement; with the arms fixed the movements are seen confined to distal portions of the upper extremities. The progressive involvement within the basal ganglia is further shown by the presence of the same form of dyskinesia in the separate parts of the lower extremities. As part of the expression of a progressive cerebral pathology, there now appears evidence of mental deterioration and an involvement of the speech mechanism, a dysarthria. This patient also showed the "Kayser-Fleischer rings".

In order to demonstrate the corneal pigmentation, the eyes of the patient showing the "Kayser-Fleischer rings" are first presented followed by a normal eye.

Cases 4 and 5—Non-identical twin sisters, 16 years of age. An exploratory laparotomy upon one of them, at the age of 13, for suspected abdominal surgical pathology disclosed a cirrhotic liver. At that time the diagnosis of hepato-lenticular degeneration was established by the further observation of the presence of Kayser-Fleischer rings and the facial expression of early Parkinsonism. The earlier pictures show the typical movements confined to small segments—index fingers—in one of the sisters. In this patient, later pictures demonstrate progressive involvement of other segments—all the fingers, both hands and beginning involvement in the legs. Early pictures of the other twin show no movements and, later, only the upper extremity involved. The Parkinsonian signs developed in progressive involvement, finally including the sympathetic nervous system—oiliness of the skin, sialorrhoea and excessive diaphoresis.

Case 6—A 57-year-old woman whose symptoms were confined to the type of dyskinesia seen in Wilson's disease. She is one of two cases shown here to illustrate hepato-lenticular degeneration occurring in later life.

At the time of observation at Montefiore Hospital, the movement was at first regarded as that of simple tremor of wide amplitude; its specific design was recognized later. The illness first appeared at about her fortieth year. All segments of the body are involved.

Case 7—This 60-year-old female patient was observed over a period of ten years. The abnormal movements involved all segments of the body, the head in greater degree. The dyskinsias, in their design, suggest a more or less irregular type of tremor. This patient came to autopsy and pathological specimens are presented here.

Pathology—A coronal section of the brain through the basal ganglia, stained for myelin sheaths, shows bilateral cavity formation in the lenticular nuclei of both sides of the brain. The liver discloses marked cirrhosis.

NEURO-OPHTHALMOLOGICAL CONDITIONS

(Film running time: 11 minutes)

A group of cases showing unusual ophthalmological conditions is presented: the pathology is essentially in the central nervous system. This group consists of patients with Marcus-Gunn phenomenon, skew deviation; various forms of monocular and binocular nystagmus; Weber's syndrome; unilateral and bilateral Duane's syndrome; myasthenia gravis, before and after prostigmin, neuromyelitis optica; congenital absence of the posterior orbital wall with pulsating enophthalmus.

Case 1—A girl, 13 years of age, shows a congenital condition in which there is an abnormal associated movement of the right upper eyelid accompanying all forms of movement of the lower jaw (Marcus-Gunn phenonemon); in repose, there is no apparent abnormality. Voluntary movements of the jaw are accompanied by automatic elevation of the right upper eyelid.

Congenital agenesis of one or more of the cranial nerves and consequent defective function or anomaly of the innervated muscles are uncommon. Congenital ptosis is not so infrequent and its presence is sometimes associated with the so-called "jaw-winking" movement. The pathological physiology is based upon abnormal structural relations in the central or peripheral nervous system involving the motor division of the fifth cranial nerve (jaw movements) and the third cranial nerve (elevation of the upper eyelid). There is no impairment of any of the ocular movements and no other defect in function of the other cranial nerves. The definite structural relationship is demonstrated by the observation that as the jaw is momentarily held in right lateral position, the associated abnormal elevation of the eyelid is synchronously maintained.

Case 2—9 years of age. This patient was operated upon and a large cerebellar neoplasm removed. Among the diagnostic classical signs was "skew deviation"; upon lateral gaze the homolateral eye turns downward and outward, the other eye synchronously upward and inward. This phenomenon occurs in brain stem lesions and its presence, with cerebellar pathology, may be secondary to compression of the brain stem; in this case, with removal of the tumor, the phenomenon disappeared. The turning of the patient's head in the picture is voluntary, due to his effort to effect monocular vision.

Case 3—46 years of age. This is the first of three cases here presented to demonstrate anomalies of nystagmus. In this patient, with disseminated sclerosis, this rather uncommon sign is observed; right lateral gaze produces a nystagmus of the right eye only and there is no nystagmus in movements of the eyes in other directions. This is due to a lesion in the brain stem affecting ascending fibers going from the nucleus of the right sixth cranial nerve to the posterior longitudinal bundle.

Case 4—41 years of age. As in the preceding patient, the classical signs of disseminated sclerosis are present. When she looks to the extreme right, a coarse mystagmus of the right eye only is produced; on gazing to the extreme left, a similar nystagmus appears, confined to the left eye. This is likewise due to a brain stem lesion, just as in the preceding instance, in the region of the sixth cranial nerve nuclei.

Case 5—Patient, 54 years of age, shows the entity, olivo-ponto-cerebellar atrophy. This rather rare condition was verified by autopsy findings. Upon left lateral gaze there is a coarse nystagmus confined to the left eye; on the right lateral and on the vertical gaze there is a binocular nystagmus. Vertical gaze is not shown on the film. Ocular involvement of this type is due to brain stem pathology, as noted in the two preceding figures.

Case 6—Patient, 59 years of age, shows a contralateral right hemiplegia with homolateral complete left third nerve paralysis (Weber's syndrome). The intact left fourth and sixth nerves maintain the eyeball in a downward and outward position as seen in the pictures. This is due to a vascular lesion in the basis pedunculi at the level of the red nucleus on the left side of the pons.

Case 7—Patient, 43 years of age, was hospitalized with the diagnosis of pernicious anemia; the neurological signs were those of subacute combined degeneration of the spinal cord. The unilateral Duane's syndrome was an incidental finding. The latter, a rarely seen entity, is a congenital condition in which there is fibrosis of the levator palpebrae superioris and of the external rectus muscles of one or both eyes. As a result, there is widening of the palpebral fissure as the eye turns laterally, and narrowing as it turns medially; there is also limitation of lateral gaze in the affected eye. The condition being of congenital origin there is no diplopia, the patient early in life learning to suppress one image. Changes of the palpebral fissures are more clearly demonstrated in the following patient.

Case 8—44 years of age. In this case, also, the findings of bilateral Duane's syndrome were incidental to her hospitalization for a condition not involving the central nervous system. The defect in both external recti muscles is of such degree that the patient is unable to rotate either eye laterally past the midline. As she looks to her left, the palpebral fissure of the left eye widens and synchronously that of the right becomes narrower; as she looks to her right, the fissure of the right eye widens with narrowing of the left.

Case 9—27 years of age, a patient with myasthenia gravis is shown in this reel to demonstrate some of the ocular phenomena seen in this disease. There is an approach to a complete external ophthalmoplegia in both eyes, to a greater degree in the left. Observe that power of convergence is lost; ptosis is more marked on the left. Pictures are also shown to demonstrate somatic involvement as is illustrated by his inability to voluntarily raise his arms repeatedly.

Pictures taken 15 minutes after the intramuscular administration of prostigmin show a pronounced improvement in power in the affected muscles. The length of time of effectiveness varies in individual cases. The influence of the drug is not sustained; however, when administered regularly, the influence is continuous. This syndrome is more fully presented in the chapter and reels on "muscular atrophies, dystrophies and allied conditions".

Case 10—39 years of age, presents sequelae of epidemic encephalitis —right hemi-paresis of extra-pyramidal origin with loss of normal associated movements of the right upper extremity. He shows the unusual phenomenon of inability to open the voluntarily closed eyes; in order to do so, he is obliged to carry out the associated movement of extreme hyperextension of the head.

Case 11—33 years of age, presents the entity, neuromyelitis optica. This disease involves the optic nerves, chiasm, and tracts and the spinal cord. In this patient vision is limited to recognition of fingers at a distance of four feet. The upper level of spinal cord involvement is evidenced by complete motor and sensory loss below the fourth dorsal dermatome. Pyramidal tract pathology is indicated by the Babinski and

Chaddock responses, and the presence of spinal reflex as shown by the involuntary spontaneous withdrawal of the paralyzed left leg, to noxious stimuli. The etiology of this condition is not known.

Case 12—42 years of age, was admitted to the Montefiore Hospital May 1943 and died in August 1943; he suffered from pulmonary and laryngeal tuberculosis. The case is of special interest with respect to the eye condition, in that such cases are rare; there was also present generalized Von Recklinghausen's disease (neuro-fibromatosis).

The following part of the family history is of interest. His father, a married sister and the latter's son and daughter also suffered from this disease.

The patient stated that there had been a ptosis of his left eyelid since birth and likewise pulsation of the eyeball. The neurofibromata are found in practically all parts of the body and varied in size.

The film presentation reveals ptosis of the left eyelid; pulsating enophthalmus on the left, synchronous with the heart beat; on pressure over the left jugular vein of the neck the eye bulges forward in a series of steps synchronous with the pulse; on coughing the eye pops violently forward into an exophthalmic position. External ocular movements can be observed limited to the internal rectus and superior oblique. The X-ray, as demonstrated on the film, shows complete absence of the posterior orbital wall; stereoscopic films reveal absence of the greater wing of the sphenoid and a small portion of the lateral part of the lesser wing. The right femur shows a chronic osteomyelitis. The loss of movement of the left eyeball is doubtless due to the congenital absence of the bony wall for the attachment of ocular muscles.

PSYCHONEUROSES

(Film running time: 16 minutes)

Organic Signs—Their Differentiation. Patients presenting signs and symptoms of seemingly psychogenic origin. The clinical syndromes show a striking similarity to those of organic pathology.

Case 1—Patient 29 years of age. The history is that of ten months of progressive weakness and stiffness of all extremities; change and fixation of facial expression; retardation of voluntary movements; posturing and loss of normal associated movements. Grossly, the picture resembles the Parkinsonian syndromes, seen as sequelae, in epidemic encephalitis. Note the apparent excessive salivation (sialorrhoea); however, there is no real salivary accumulation and drooling. Careful observation discloses voluntary facial and jaw movements, with retained saliva, through which air is being blown by the patient; one might easily overlook this important point in differential diagnosis, also the bizarre fixed postures of fingers and left foot. The symptoms included marked personality changes, emotional instability, at times negativism and evidences of psychic withdrawal from his immediate environment; in some moments he was entirely inaccessible to contact with the examiners. His subjective complaints included mild somatic delusions and with these he assumed a marked invalidism. Psychological difficulties and emotional stress in his domestic situation were obviously related to the onset and development of the illness.

The patient is first shown as he appeared on admission. Psychotherapy, including hypnosis, was instituted at that time and continued over a period of four weeks. During the brief periods of hypnosis and intensive suggestion, the symptoms were removed and the treatment finally induced essentially complete restoration to his normal state. Pictures of the patient at this time are shown; rigidity, posturing, anomaly of salivation and fixation in facial expression are no longer present. He is now mentally alert and responsive.

Following discontinuance of all treatment for three weeks, the abnormal clinical picture recurred; the patient is again shown as he was at this period. Of much interest and bearing upon the nature of the group of patients, illustrating the theme in this set of films, is the progressive development of this case. Psychotic behavior and apparent fixation of the somatic signs made it necessary later to place the patient in a psychiatric hospital. A final diagnosis of schizophrenia-catatonic type and with added paranoid trends, gives added interest to the original picture.

Case 2—An unmarried woman of 29. The immediate precipitating cause of her illness was an emotional upset associated with the marriage of her brother. The physical signs of this psychogenic state, as demonstrated in the pictures, were voluntary persistent forced closure of the eyes with strong resistance to all efforts to open them actively or passively. The peculiar posturing of the fingers and the type of tremor suggest its psychogenic nature; they are not seen in organic disease. Efforts to help the patient stand and walk emphasize the bizarre forms of posture and movements seen in cases of psychogenic origin; the gait is that of astasia abasia.

Case 3—44 years of age. The patient may be said to represent a somatic symbolic response to wishful thinking. This married woman, though ardently desiring motherhood, had never conceived. She also had some mild psychosomatic symptoms. The irregular, periodic symbolization of pregnancy appears in the form of a sudden enlargement of the abdomen (pseudocyesis), attaining in its size and contour the dimensions of a full term pregnancy; this occurred spontaneously but could likewise be induced by pressure over the right upper abdominal quadrant. This bizarre physical phenomenon would continue for a variable time, usually a few minutes; it would spontaneously and gradually recede. The abnormal contour of the abdominal wall was attended by a peculiar posturing of the fingers of the left hand with a strong resistance to change in their configuration. The physiological basis of this mechanism is conjectural.

Case 4—A previously healthy individual, 29 years of age; immediately following an industrial trauma involving litigation, the symptoms shown in the following clinical picture appeared. There are episodes of apparent unconsciousness with easily recognized evidences of voluntary control and efforts at resistance. Personality changes characterize and give color to the clinical setting. The emotional factor is visualized in the facial distortions and attitudes of the patient.

The localized, functional convulsive movements of the left upper extremity are brought to momentary cessation by the forced extension of the left forearm by the examiner. Localized convulsive seizures, with distortions, could be induced by simple and sudden physical stimulus, for example, grasping the patient's forearm. The pictures throughout are clearly defined, as of psychogenic origin; they conform to no recognized organic pathology.

Case 5—54 years of age, was observed over a period of six years. The first pictures show the patient shortly after a fall from a ladder not resulting in evident physical injury. The symptoms appeared suddenly and were at that time regarded as of purely psychogenic nature; they included definite emotional effects. Among the motor manifestations, one sees bizarre response in the finger to nose test and the abnormal gait—seemingly a form of "astasia abasia". The design, however, is that of "marche a petits pas" and suggests organic disease. The latter symptoms occurred only after the patient had been in a ward, in which there were patients with multiple sclerosis showing marked organic signs, which the patient seems to be imitating. Among the earlier symptoms were changes in behavior suggestive of conversion hysteria; his conduct was silly, with labile, superficial emotions. He was discharged from the hospital with the diagnosis of psychoneurosis, conversion hysteria. About four years later he returned to Montefiore Hospital showing essentially the same symptoms but in an aggravated form. The man died of bronchopneumonia. On post-mortem examination, the brain presented the histopathological picture typical of encephalopathia periaxialis diffusa (Schilder's Disease). Myelin sheath preparations are shown in the films; one observes preservation of the arcuate fibers of the cortex with demyelinization of the fibers of the centrum ovale. Thus, in this instance, an apparently psychogenic picture was based upon an organic pathology. One may theorize upon the subtle question of the origin and relationship in the development of the clinical signs and symptoms—were the signs and symptoms originally organic or psychogenic?

Case 6—A woman 34 years of age, unmarried, is shown in the supine position to secure patient's relaxation. The essential clinical picture is that of tremors limited to the left upper and right lower extremities. The tempo and design of the tremor in the left arm and right leg are not the same. There is no increase in tone. The tremors, while rhythmical, change in form and design upon volitional movements of the affected extremities as well as other segments of the body. The right foot tends to dystonic posture; the left to the psychogenic posture of maintained plantar flexion of the toes in the absence of muscular involvement. The clinical picture approximates that of chronic encephalitis but is of psychogenic etiology.

PSYCHONEUROSES

Case 7—63 years of age, has been under observation at the Montefiore Hospital for 26 years. The diagnosis of the functional character of the condition was made upon admission and the clinical picture remained the same until death. There were no organic signs at any time and no psychotic features. She is seen here in a posture (Buddha) which did not change materially during the entire time of her hospitalization. Observation has never revealed voluntary movement in her lower extremities; the absence of muscular atrophy is one of the striking features. Patient developed bronchopneumonia and died. Careful post-mortem studies, gross and microscopic, showed no pathological changes of nerve structure. A small meningioma, size of a pea, was found in the cerebral dura in the region of the central fissure on the right side. It gave no signs or symptoms. One may think of a catatonic type of reaction.

Case 8—51 years of age. The history reveals a definite relationship between the onset of his illness and recent domestic difficulties; organic neurological signs are absent. Patient is first shown seated. There is apparent defect in voluntary power and control in essentially all groups of muscles; he appears to be unable to raise his arms above the horizontal; there is a bizarre type of movement in all extremities. In walking, the same form of disturbed motility is seen; it is a type of "astasia abasia". In all the pictures of the patient, the movements in their magnitude approach convulsive degree. In the supine position, the movements are seen in greater intensity and in design and force closely approach organic convulsive seizures; there is no impairment of consciousness. Patient was given a course of ten metrazol injections and is shown while receiving the fourth and the fifth. The anticipated organic convulsive seizure immediately follows each of the injections. With the return of consciousness following each treatment, the abnormal movements ceased for a time and, following the fifth injection, there was apparent return to normalcy. The mental attitude of the patient, one of depression and emotional instability during his illness, is now that of his former normal state. The final pictures show the patient entirely restored. Our period of observation covers about six months.

SOMATIC ENDOCRINE TYPES

(Film running time: 15 minutes)

Patients demonstrating various somatic endocrine syndromes, namely: dyschondroplastic dwarfism, achondroplastic dwarfism, acromegalic giantism, pituitary (Froehlich) syndrome, pituitary-pineal syndrome, hermaphroditism, Lawrence-Moon-Biedl syndrome, dysdactylism, cretinism, albinism, mongolism, microcephalus and hydrocephalus.

Case 1—A dyschondroplastic dwarf, 29 years of age, of Italian ancestry. She is a mental defective with an intelligence quotient of 41 and was small and cyanotic at birth. She had rickets in infancy, was retarded in physical development and gained only very slowly in weight. Dentition began at 11 months; she walked and talked at one year and physical growth practically ceased at four years.

Though miniature in physical stature at ·this time, there is no disproportion in segmental development; the relationship between the various segments of the trunk and the extremities, is normal. There is uniform involvement of all bony structures. This condition is due to a congenital defect of the cartilaginous bones.

This patient is moody, emotionally unstable and altogether a behavior problem. However, she is capable of doing fine handwork and ordinary housework.

Case 2—An achondroplastic dwarf, 30 years of age, of Irish ancestry. He is a mental defective with an intelligence quotient of 77. At birth the patient was observed to have an unusualy large head. He walked in his fifth and talked in his sixth year. His growth ceased at about that period.

Observe the dwarfed stature and, in this case, the segmental disproportion. The trunk and head are of normal adult size; the relative disproportions in length between the several segments of the extremities (arm to forearm, thigh to leg) are striking. The arms and legs are very short; the hands are of trident type. Observe the anomalous distribution of hair; it is limited to the lower two-thirds of the legs below the knees. It ends abruptly, like a collar, and there is no hair on the thighs. There is a peculiar localized muscle contour, just below the elbow, demonstrated as the hand is voluntarily flexed and extended. This condition

SOMATIC ENDOCRINE TYPES

is a result of a congenital defect of the cartilaginous bones.

The patient is active and productive as a printer. He is good natured, contented, and presents no behavior problems.

Case 3—An acromegalic giant, 25 years of age. He is a mental defective with an intelligence quotient of 36. His father was an alcoholic. At six months of age and continuing up to the present, convulsive seizures of undetermined etiology have been observed. Dentition occurred at one year, he walked at three and talked at four. Unusually large stature was observed during his first decade.

He had an approximately normal length of trunk, but abnormally long extremities, hands and feet. In the demonstration, examiner's hand and foot are displayed for contrast. Patient is a classical example of pituitary dysfunction.

Cases 4, 5 and 6—A group of three patients demonstrating Froehlich's Syndrome is presented. From left to right the patients are as follows:

A mental defective, 26 years of age, whose intelligence quotient is 61, is of Roumanian ancestry. It is of interest to note that the mother suffered from multiple lipomatosis; there is otherwise no relevant factor in the family history. Birth and delivery were normal although the patient weighed 16 pounds. Dentition occurred at 9 months; she walked and talked at two years. From her fifth to her seventh years, she suffered from seizures said to have been "fainting attacks". She started school at six and at 13 had reached only the second grade; she was then demoted to an ungraded class. Patient was treated in various hospitals for obesity; she has always been quarrelsome, unruly and careless in personal care and appearance.

A mental defective, 21 years of age, whose intelligence quotient is 44, is of Irish-Canadian ancestry. Her family history is essentially free from taint. Though only four pounds in weight at birth, delivery was difficult, a breech presentation and instrumental. She walked and talked at three years; entered kindergarten at six years but was soon removed because of mental deficiency.

A mental defective, 32 years of age, with an intelligence quotient of 56. Both parents and her siblings were mentally defective; her father was an alcoholic. Birth was normal; she talked at two and walked at four years. She entered school at eight but could not go beyond the third grade.

In the pictures, observe in all three patients the pendulous quilt of adipose tissue over the abdomen; this is more evident in the lateral views. In the posterior view, as they stand together one sees a marked difference in circumferences in the lower extremities in each of the two end patients. To demonstrate the disproportionately small feet and hands, the feet of one patient are shown. Observe the extensive varicosities and fat deposits in the lower extremities. A lateral view of patient on the right visualizes the ponderous adiposity with the voluminous and pendulous breasts. Note on posterior view the contour of fat formation on the trunk under the right shoulder creating the illusion of a misplaced mammary gland.

In all these cases, one observes excessive deposits of fat around the hips, abdomen and shoulders; the fat is found more particularly in the proximal rather than distal parts of the extremities. Fingers taper to unusually small tips. The large breasts are due to subcutaneous fat and not to increase of glandular tissue. As illustrated in the next case shown, there is hypogenitalia in the male. This metabolic dyscrasia is due to pathology in the central nervous system (hypothalamus) and in the pituitary gland.

Case 7—A mental defective, 27 years of age, whose intelligence quotient is 42, presents the syndrome as seen in the male. He weighed 11 pounds at birth, talked at two and walked at three years. There is nothing relevant in the family history.

In full view, the patient's general contour suggests female configuration. The adiposity is evident and its disposition is essentially as in the female. Note the gonadal underdevelopment.

Cases 8, 9 and 10—A group of three patients, demonstrating the pituitary-pineal syndrome, is presented. From left to right, the patients are as follows:

A mental defective, 27 years of age, is now classed as an idiot. She was able to complete grammar grades. Birth was normal but marked hirsutism of body and face was observed at that time. She walked and talked at fifteen months. At the age of three, she suffered an illness said to have been erysipelas, followed by developmental change. Epileptiform seizures, beginning in her seventh year, have continued up to the present. She is inactive, seclusive and unreliable, with violent outbursts of temper.

A mental defective, 37 years of age, of Russian ancestry, whose intelligence quotient is 28. The family history is entirely free from taint. Patient's birth was normal; she walked at 18 months and began to talk at three years, but language, both in content and expression, remained underdeveloped. She attended school at eight but only for a brief period because of mental deficiency. Between 12 and 16 she became obese but remained short in stature; later she lost markedly in weight.

A mental defective, 32 years of age, of German ancestry whose intelligence quotient is ten. The record of the paternal ancestry is pertinent; it includes three psychotic individuals and one uncle who was deaf and dumb. Patient, born at term, was instrumentally delivered. She walked at two and talked at three years. The only infectious disease noted was measles in her second year. Her intellectual defect and abnormal behavior precluded her attendance at school.

In the pictures, observe that the two end subjects show the classical distribution of adipose tissue of the Froehlich syndrome (as shown in the preceding group). It is of interest to note that the physical configuration of the patient in the middle had changed in later years; pronounced adiposity which developed between the ages of 12 and 16 gradually disappeared. In addition, these patients present anomalous hirsuties, the location of which is characteristic of the male. Both the hirsuties and the configuration of head and face give a masculine appearance to these patients. The syndrome suggests pathology in both pituitary and pineal glands and the adrenals also may be implicated.

Case 11—31 years of age, is of normal intelligence. Other than diabetes in father and sister, family history offers nothing pertinent. Her husband suffered from paresis, symptoms of which appeared three years after marriage. Patient was never pregnant. She rapidly became blind, the result of optic atrophy; there was paresis of all the external ocular muscles and deafness in the left ear, probably of central origin. There was partial transmutation from female to male somatic character. The clitoris became markedly hypertrophied and the patient developed a male facial contour with male type of hair distribution on the face. At about this period, there was an episode of temporary mental confusion with disorientation and euphoria. The pathological localization is probably the same as that in the three previous patients. Lues may have been a basic factor.

Case 12—A mental defective, 16 years of age, with an intelligence quotient of 37, comes from a family with definite taint, including lues, alcomolism, mental deficiency and prostitution. Patient presents the picture of hermaphroditism. Except for the dysplasia of the genitalia there is nothing pertinent in his somatic development.

Observe the absence of pubic hair. Testis is present only on the right. The structural relationship between the penis and what corresponds to the scrotum suggests that of clitoris and labia majora. Just below the penis one sees a small vulva and introitus.

Case 13—A mental defective, 19 years of age, whose intelligence quotient is 55, presents the classical clinical picture of the Lawrence-Moon-Biedl Syndrome. There is a history of insanity and tuberculosis in the immediate progenitors; father and mother were first cousins. Patient born at full term, spontaneous delivery, dentition at five months, walked at one and one half years and talked at two years of age. Amaurosis began at two and has progressed to a degree where sight is limited to a very small area of peripheral vision. Obesity was first observed in patient's eighth year and, at about the same period, a tendency to rapid fatiguability; polyuria and polydypsia began at about the same time. The clinical picture now includes bilateral retinitis pigmentosa, marked adiposity, especially at the pelvic girdle and in the breasts, syndactylism and polydactylism, microgenitalia, undescended right testicle and female distribution of pubic hair.

The first pictures show uncertainty of gait because of visual defect and is likewise demonstrated when the patient attempts to follow the moving finger placed within a few inches of his eyes; this test also demonstrates paresis of the external ocular muscles. The hypogonadal development, abdominal adiposity and female distribution of pubic hair are visualized. The polydactylism (six fingers in the right hand) and the bilateral syndactylism are demonstrated. The tendency to syndactylism is also present in the feet. In addition to the obvious degenerative features, there is a polyglandular dyscrasia (pituitary, testis and possibly adrenal).

Case 14—A mental defective, 18 years of age, of Greek ancestry, with an intelligence quotient of 55, is a case of dysdactylism, "claw-hands" and "claw-feet". No other structural anomalies are present in the family history. He was a full-term child, weighing 14 pounds. The deformities were observed at birth. Dentition occurred at ten months, he walked at 18 months and talked at about three years. He appreciates and is sensitive of his deformities; quiet, affable, obedient, he offers no behavior problem. Despite the deformities, he possesses some degree of manual dexterity.

The pictures show that the defects are much the same in form in both hands. The feet, also involved, show structural anomalies strikingly similar in form to those observed in the hands, but in lesser degree.

Case 15—A cretin, 25 years of age, of Austrian ancestry, with myxedema; his intelligence quotient is 45. Family history is irrelevant. He walked and talked at about three years of age. Early in life patient was given thyroid without apparent influence upon his condition. He presents the features of of myxedema—thick edematous lips and eyelids, baggy cheeks, wrinkled forehead, base of nose broad, hair coarse, scanty and dry, skin thickened, dry and scaly, and a protuberant abdomen.

Case 16—A mental defective, 37 years of age, with an intelligence quotient of 14, is another cretin who has an unusually large thyroid adenoma. Her personal and family history have not been available for survey.

The typical somatic features of cretinism are seen in the pictures, although thyroid of such size and contour is unusual.

Case 17—A mental defective, 34 years of age, of Italian ancestry, with an intelligence quotient of 47, shows the somatic features of albinism. Development in childhood was normal; at 17 he was placed in an institution for the blind because of progressive amaurosis. Albinism, of course, is not necessarily attended by mental deficiency. Among his three siblings, two are albinos. Albinism is of heredo-familial nature; the somatic biological defect is based upon a deficiency in pigment in the skin, hair and retinae.

In the pictures, note the absence of pigment in the hair of the head and in the pubic region; the hair is pure white.

Case 18 and 19—Brothers, of Italian ancestry, 24 and 27 years of age respectively, each with an intelligence quotient of 17. They are Mongolian idiots. Mental deficiency was observed in infancy. The physical characteristics associated with Mongolian idiocy are demonstrated in the subjects presented. Observe the obliquity of the lid-slits and the peculiar countenance resembling the facies of the Mongol race.

In these cases, the brain is usually below average size and is structurally characterized by simplified cortical and vascular patterns.

Case 20—A mental defective, 22 years of age, of Russian ancestry, with an intelligence quotient of 18, is another example of Mongolism. An unusual feature in this case is the macroglossia, made especially evident upon protrusion of the huge tongue.

Case 21—A mental defective, 14 years of age, of West Indian ancestry, with an intelligence quotient of 10, is an example of Mongolism, a condition rarely observed in the colored race. He presents the classical features outlined above.

Cases 22 and 23—Brothers, 18 and 21 years of age respectively, of

Italian ancestry, are mental defectives with intelligence quotient of 30 and 40 respectively. They are microcephalic.

These cases present the characteristic small head of peculiar contour with recessive forehead. In such cases, the fontanelles may be prematurely cloesd.

Post-mortem examination in cases of microcephaly discloses a small brain (usually less than 1000 grams in weight); its general appearance in gross structure suggests a low stage of development in the human scale.

Case 24—A mental defective, 10 years of age, of Italian ancestry, with an intelligence quotient of 15, is another illustration of microcephaly. The head at birth was observed to be unusually small. Although dentition and walking occurred in the first year, patient never talked.

Case 25, 26, and 27—A group of three patients, showing hydrocephalus, is presented. From left to right, they are:

1. A mental defective 9 years of age, of German-Italian ancestry, with an intelligence quotient of 54. The patient's head began to grow rapidly during the first months of life. He had rickets; convulsions occurred during his second year.

2. A mental defective, 6 years of age, of Danish-Irish ancestry, with an intelligence quotient of 21. The diagnosis of hydrocephalus was made at birth.

3. A mental defective, 11 years of age, of French-Irish ancestry, with an intelligence quotient of 40. He was a premature infant born at seven months by instrumental delivery. Abnormally large head was first observed at nine months.

The cranial enlargement in the majority of these cases is due to increased cerebro-spinal fluid pressure. The head enlargement is more or less uniform, though most marked in the antero-posterior diameter, with protrusion of the frontal bones, as seen in the cases presented.

ENCEPHALOGRAPHIC STUDIES IN EXTRAPYRAMIDAL DISEASES

(This film deals predominantly with changes in the ventricular system; it is not intended to demonstrate clinical entities.)

(Film running time: 9 minutes)

In this reel we are presenting groups of cases with their corresponding encephalograms. The purpose of these studies is to demonstrate the relationship between the clinical and the anatomical pathology, with especial reference to the ventricular system and its relationship to the anatomical centers involved. The groups shown are chronic degenerative chorea, progressive hepato-lenticular degeneration, dystonia musculorum deformans, Little's disease and double athetosis. In each case antero-posterior and lateral views are presented. Some of these patients, without accompanying encephalograms, are included in other reels.

Analyses of the individual clinical pictures are omitted here; they are outlined in the respective reels in which the specific entities are presented.

Case 1—49 years of age. Chronic degenerative chorea (Huntington type). 175 cc. spinal fluid removed; 170 cc. air injected. There is symmetrical bilateral ventricular dilatation; third and fourth ventricles and aqueduct are somewhat dilated; moderately severe bilateral cortical atrophy.

Case 2—44 years of age. Chronic degenerative chorea (Huntington's type). 180 cc. spinal fluid removed; 175 cc. air injected. There is moderate bilateral ventricular dilatation, right greater than left; third and fourth ventricles and aqueduct dilated; moderately severe cortical atrophy involving superior temporal, supramarginal, angular, middle and inferior gyri and Island of Reil.

Case 3—34 years of age. Chronic degenerative chorea (Huntington's type). Father suffered from the same disease. The illness, in the patient presented, began at the unusually early age of 27. The mental symptoms appeared a few years after the first physical signs. Psychometric studies disclosed a mental age of 7 years, 8 months. 165 cc. spinal fluid removed; 160 cc. air injected. Encephalograms show moderate bilateral dilatation of both lateral ventricles, right greater than left, involving predominantly frontal horns and the anterior third of the bodies of the lateral ventricles; third and fourth ventricles and aqueduct are slightly dilated; moderately severe bilateral cortical atrophy.

Case 4—22 years of age. Progressive hepato-lenticular degeneration. 165 cc. spinal fluid removed; 160 cc. air injected. Frontal horns and anterior portion of bodies of lateral ventricles and fourth ventricle are dilated; bilateral cortical atrophy of the precentral and premotor areas.

Cases 5 and 6—Non-identical twins, 16 years of age. Progressive hepato-lenticular degeneration. 127 cc. spinal fluid removed; 120 cc. air injected. In both cases, anterior portions of both lateral ventricles are dilated; pictures are otherwise normal.

Case 7—17 years of age. Idiopathic dystonia musculorum deformans. 160 cc. spinal fluid removed; 150 cc. air injected. Except for slight dilatation of the third ventricle, encephalograms are normal.

Case 8—14 years of age. Idiopathic dystonia musculorum deformans. 115 cc. spinal fluid removed, 110 cc. air injected. Encephalograms are normal.

Case 9—43 years of age. Dystonia musculorum deformans, static type. Four months after an injury, accompanied by unconsciousness, at the age of 20, the dyskinesias began and were progressive; at 27, postures became static and fixed. 320 cc. of spinal fluid were removed; 300 cc. air were injected. Generalized cortical atrophy with coarse sulci; the ventricular system is not dilated. The enormous amount of fluid present was due to the external hydrocephalus.*

Case 10—37 years of age. Little's disease; "double athetosis". 173 cc. spinal fluid removed; 168 cc. air injected. Encephalograms are normal. This is compatible with the type of minute pathology found in this type of extrapyramidal disease—status marmoratus and status dysmyelinisatus —in which there is no gross distortion of the ventricular system.

Case 11—31 years of age. Little's disease, congenital spastic triplegia. 180 cc. spinal fluid removed; 175 cc. air injected. Large area of porencephaly in right frontal area; bilateral internal hydrocephalus; cortical atrophy.

---

* Putnam has observed a perhaps distinctive encephalographic abnormality in cases of athetosis and dystonia, namely: a depression of the floor of the body of the lateral ventricle out of proportion to the dilatation. The condition is suggested in several of our cases.

APPENDIX

The following films, for which this manual provides supplementary text, are available from the New York University Film Library, 71 Washington Square South, New York 12, New York.

Chorea.—Gives brief outline of the three groups of chronic degenerative chorea: Huntington, arteriosclerotic and post encephalitic. (See pp. 1-4)

Film running time: 10 minutes. $2.00 a day; sale $25.00.

Convulsive and Allied Conditions.—Patients demonstrating the following disorders are shown: Maladie des tics; generalized myoclonic movements following acute epidemic encephalitis; myoclonus epilepsy (Unverricht); palatal myoclonus; catalepsy; narcolepsy associated with cataplexy; convulsive state in hypoglycemia; Jacksonian seizures (due to cerebral neoplasm); convulsions of psychogenic origin. (See pp. 5-7)

Film running time: 11 minutes. $2.00 a day; sale $25.00.

Dystonia Musculorum Deformans.—Patients suffering from various forms of dystonia are depicted. One patient is shown in various phases of her illness, observed over a period of some seventeen years. The case was originally diagnosed as psychogenic. (See pp. 8-18)

Film running time: 20 minutes. $3.50 a day; sale $45.00.

Epidemic Encephalitis.—Each case presents some particular feature of the sequelae of epidemic encephalitis. Diagnostic values are stressed. These graphic visualizations present sequential histories in most cases over a period of years of observation. Some very bizarre entities are demonstrated. (See pp. 19-26)

Film running time: 19 minutes. $3.50 a day; sale $45.00.

Friedreich's Hereditary Ataxia and Little's Disease.—Four cases of hereditary ataxia are visually demonstrated—two brothers and two sisters showing classical signs of this entity. Cases of Little's Disease are presented showing various forms of dyskinesias of congenital origin. The abnormal movements are predominantly of extrapyramidal type. (See pp. 27-30)

Film running time: 10 minutes. $2.00 a day; sale $25.00.

APPENDIX

Progressive Muscular Atrophies, Dystrophies and Allied Conditions.—Illustrative cases are given for each of the above groups. Distinctive diagnostic features are pointed out. (See pp. 31-41)

Film running time: 15 minutes. $3.50 a day; sale $40.00.

Progressive Hepato-Lenticular Degeneration.—Patients are shown demonstrating the various neurological signs of entities involving brain and liver pathology. The cerebral lesions are in the extrapyramidal system. (See pp. 42-45)

Film running time: 9 minutes. $2.00 a day; sale $25.00.

Neuro-Ophthalmological Conditions: Pathological Ocular Manifestations of Clinical Interest.—Abnormal neurological conditions associated with pathological signs relating to vision are demonstrated. (See pp. 46-49)

Film running time: 11 minutes. $2.00 a day; sale $25.00.

Psychoneuroses.—Patients are demonstrated presenting signs and symptoms of seemingly psychogenic nature. However, they also show clinical syndromes suggestive of organic disease. Differential diagnosis is considered. (See pp. 50-53)

Film running time: 16 minutes. $3.50 a day; sale $40.00.

Somatic Endocrine Types.—The groups demonstrated are dyschondroplastic dwarfism, acromegalic giantism, pituitary (Froelich) syndrome, pituitary-pineal syndrome, hermaphroditism, Lawrence-Moon-Biedl syndrome, dysdactylism, cretinism, albinism, Mongolism, micro and hydrocephalus. (See pp. 54-60)

Film running time: 15 minutes. $3.50 a day; sale $40.00.

Encephalographic Studies in Extrapyramidal Diseases.—This reel demonstrates changes in the ventricular system and is not intended to demonstrate clinical entities. (See pp. 61-62)

Film running time: 9 minutes. $2.00 a day; sale $25.00.